Recent Clinical Advances in Cardiac Rehabilitation

Recent Clinical Advances in Cardiac Rehabilitation

Guest Editor

Tomasz Rechciński

MDPI • Basel • Beijing • Wuhan • Barcelona • Belgrade • Novi Sad • Cluj • Manchester

Guest Editor
Tomasz Rechciński
1st Department of Cardiology
Medical University of Lodz
Lodz
Poland

Editorial Office
MDPI AG
Grosspeteranlage 5
4052 Basel, Switzerland

This is a reprint of the Special Issue, published open access by the journal *Journal of Clinical Medicine* (ISSN 2077-0383), freely accessible at: https://www.mdpi.com/journal/jcm/special_issues/0F0KSN4C09.

For citation purposes, cite each article independently as indicated on the article page online and as indicated below:

Lastname, A.A.; Lastname, B.B. Article Title. *Journal Name* **Year**, *Volume Number*, Page Range.

ISBN 978-3-7258-8265-6 (Hbk)
ISBN 978-3-7258-8266-3 (PDF)
https://doi.org/10.3390/books978-3-7258-8266-3

Contents

About the Editor

Tomasz Rechciński

Tomasz Rechciński, MD, PhD, DSc, is a cardiologist, academic teacher and clinical researcher based in Łódź, Poland. He is affiliated with the Department of Cardiology of the Medical University of Lodz and is also engaged in everyday work at a cardiac rehabilitation unit, a combination that allows his academic interests to remain closely connected to the realities of patient care and secondary prevention.

Over the years, his professional interests have focused on cardiac rehabilitation, long-term cardiovascular prevention and the care of patients after acute coronary syndromes and coronary interventions. His work has included studies on exercise capacity and rehabilitation outcomes in patients with incomplete revascularisation, publications on the evolving role of modern rehabilitation and telerehabilitation in contemporary cardiology, and clinical papers reflecting a broader commitment to bringing evidence-based cardiovascular care closer to daily practice.

What links his clinical and academic activity is a lasting conviction that cardiac rehabilitation should be practical, grounded in solid evidence and firmly rooted in the real lives of patients. He has long valued the multidisciplinary nature of this field and the contribution of physicians, physiotherapists, psychologists, dietitians and other health professionals who help patients regain confidence and function after a cardiac event.

Preface

Cardiac rehabilitation has travelled a long way from its cautious beginnings as a selective intervention for patients recovering from myocardial infarction. Today, it is recognised as one of the foundations of secondary prevention: a multidimensional process that combines exercise training, optimisation of medical therapy, lifestyle counselling, psychological care and support for a meaningful return to everyday life. Yet despite strong evidence and clear recommendations, rehabilitation remains underused, unevenly implemented and too often perceived as an adjunct rather than an integral part of cardiovascular treatment.

The entries gathered in this volume originate from a Special Issue of the *Journal of Clinical Medicine* devoted to recent clinical advances in cardiac rehabilitation. Read together, they show a field that is mature in its principles, but still evolving in its practice. The authors, representing centres from Europe, Africa and Asia, do not merely summarise current knowledge; they portray a discipline responding to new technologies, new patient needs and new expectations regarding long-term, person-centred cardiovascular care.

Several contributions revisit questions that remain surprisingly unresolved: who is referred to rehabilitation, who actually attends, and why so many patients still do not receive the support that guidelines clearly endorse. Others focus on hybrid and technology-assisted models of care, accelerated by the COVID-19 pandemic, showing that rehabilitation can remain safe, effective and meaningful even when it extends beyond the traditional hospital setting. These innovations do not replace the human core of rehabilitation; if used wisely, they may help more people reach it.

A particular strength of this Reprint is the breadth of its intended audience. It is addressed not only to cardiologists, internists and physicians involved in rehabilitation medicine, but also to psychologists, physiotherapists, dietitians and nurses whose expertise is indispensable to genuinely multidisciplinary care. It may also speak to researchers in exercise physiology and related basic and translational sciences, since several entries remind us that the benefits of rehabilitation can be understood at many levels—from motivation, family support and behaviour change to mitochondrial energetics and cellular responses to training.

This wide perspective is not accidental. Cardiac rehabilitation has never been solely about supervised exercise sessions or discharge recommendations. At its best, it is a way of helping people recover not only physical capacity, but also confidence, rhythm, autonomy and a sense of future after a major cardiovascular event. That is why the psychological, social and family dimensions running through many of the chapters feel as important as the clinical and physiological ones.

Another notable feature of this collection is its attention to patients who are often less visible in the usual rehabilitation narrative. Women, older adults, patients with heart failure, individuals with unusual arrhythmic syndromes and those facing practical or emotional barriers to participation appear here not as marginal cases, but as people whose experiences challenge us to make rehabilitation more flexible, more inclusive and more faithful to real life. If cardiac rehabilitation is to fulfil its promise, it must be capable of fitting not only diagnoses and recommendations, but also the everyday circumstances in which recovery actually unfolds.

For clinicians, this volume offers thoughtful and practical perspectives on how rehabilitation can be delivered in a changing world. For allied health professionals, it affirms that effective rehabilitation is built on collaboration rather than hierarchy. For scientists, it points toward questions that remain open and still deserve careful study. And for everyone engaged in cardiovascular care, it carries a simple message: rehabilitation is not an optional addition to treatment, but one of its most effective and most human forms.

It is hoped that the entries collected here will serve not only as a record of current knowledge but also as an invitation to think more broadly about what cardiac rehabilitation can become. If this Reprint encourages even a few readers to design better programmes, ask better questions or reach patients who might otherwise be overlooked, it will already have achieved something worthwhile.

Tomasz Rechciński
Guest Editor

Journal of
Clinical Medicine

MDPI

Editorial

Cardiac Rehabilitation in 2026: Bridging Guideline Mandates, Patient Realities and Emerging Innovations

Tomasz Rechciński [1,*], Barbara Bralewska [2] and Aleksandra Rechcińska [3]

1 1st Department of Cardiology, Medical University of Lodz, 91-347 Lodz, Poland
2 SP ZOZ Central Clinical Hospital, Medical University of Lodz, 92-213 Lodz, Poland
3 Independent Researcher, 90-014 Lodz, Poland
* Correspondence: tomasz.rechcinski@office365.umed.pl

We are pleased to introduce the Special Issue of the Journal of Clinical Medicine, dedicated to "Recent Clinical Advances in Cardiac Rehabilitation", which addresses one of the most critical topics in secondary prevention of cardiovascular diseases.

In the Brothers Grimm's timeless fairy tale, a prince trapped in the body of a frog awaits a single transformative kiss to reclaim his true form. Cardiac rehabilitation has long resembled this enchanted prince: a therapy with royal evidence behind it, yet still confined to a marginal, often overlooked place in routine care. What it now awaits is not magic, but the deliberate "kiss" of full implementation—across regions, cultures and health systems—that would finally allow its true potential to emerge.

Contemporary guidelines from both Europe and Asia leave little doubt about the central role of cardiac rehabilitation in secondary prevention. The 2021 ESC Guidelines on cardiovascular disease prevention in clinical practice explicitly position structured rehabilitation as a core component of integrated risk-factor management, lifestyle modification and long-term follow-up after major cardiovascular events [1]. Similarly, consensus recommendations from Japanese expert groups emphasise that every patient after myocardial infarction should be offered a comprehensive, multidisciplinary rehabilitation programme, combining exercise training, education, psychological support and vocational counselling as a standard of care rather than a luxury [2]. Together, these documents set a clear, global benchmark: high-quality cardiac rehabilitation is no longer optional—it is a clinical imperative.

Yet, as so often in cardiovascular prevention, what is written in guidelines is not what patients receive in everyday practice. Recent data from the INTERASPIRE programme paint a sobering picture of secondary prevention and cardiac rehabilitation worldwide, showing that a large proportion of patients with established coronary heart disease are neither referred to, nor enrolled in, structured rehabilitation, and that achievement of lifestyle and risk-factor targets remains disappointingly low. Despite robust evidence and strong recommendations, many patients leave hospital without a clear path towards sustained physical activity, smoking cessation, weight control or psychosocial support [3].

Reports from China echo this paradox in a rapidly transforming healthcare system. Although the epidemiological burden of cardiovascular disease is immense and awareness of secondary prevention is growing, participation in supervised exercise-based rehabilitation and long-term adherence to lifestyle changes remain limited, mirroring the global pattern of underuse and unmet need [4]. In both international and national registries, the gap between the "ideal world" of guidelines and the "real world" of practice is striking—and it is this gap that continues to keep cardiac rehabilitation in its frog-like state, far from the royal status it deserves.

The COVID-19 pandemic unexpectedly acted as a stress test—and, paradoxically, as an accelerator—for cardiac rehabilitation. When centre-based programmes were abruptly interrupted or severely restricted, clinicians and patients were forced to experiment with new ways of delivering exercise training, education and psychosocial support at a distance. This disruption revealed how fragile our reliance on in-person models had been, but it also highlighted the adaptability of rehabilitation when digital tools, telemonitoring and home-based protocols are embraced [5].

In this context, several contributions in the present Special Issue offer concrete examples of how innovation can preserve—and sometimes even enhance—access to rehabilitation despite structural barriers. One study explores a structured telerehabilitation pathway that combines remote supervision, education and regular feedback to maintain exercise intensity and adherence in high-risk patients who cannot attend traditional centre-based programmes (Contributor 1). Another article examines hybrid models that blend on-site assessments with technology-assisted home sessions, showing that such approaches can sustain functional gains and risk-factor control while reducing travel burden and improving convenience (Contributor 2). Together, these works suggest that the pandemic may have been the long-awaited external shock that pushed cardiac rehabilitation closer to the transformative "kiss" of technology-enabled care.

Beyond simple telemonitoring and video visits, more technologically advanced models are beginning to emerge. A recent study on technology-assisted cardiac rehabilitation in patients with coronary heart disease, for example, integrates wearable sensors, mobile applications and structured remote coaching into a cohesive programme that delivers supervised exercise, behavioural support and risk-factor management outside the walls of the hospital. Such interventions move beyond emergency solutions and start to define a new standard of care in which digital tools are not a temporary substitute, but an integral layer of rehabilitation delivery [6].

The notion that cardiac rehabilitation can be "augmented" rather than merely "reproduced" by technology resonates strongly with the themes of this Special Issue. By systematically embedding monitoring, feedback and personalised adjustment into patients' daily lives, higher-level technological solutions may help address long-standing problems of adherence, equity and scalability. The question is no longer whether technology can support rehabilitation, but how to design, evaluate and implement these programmes so that their benefits reach the patients who need them most

At the same time, cardiac rehabilitation must widen its gaze beyond the "typical" post-myocardial infarction or post-revascularisation patient. Emerging evidence underscores the needs of groups that have historically been underrepresented in programmes and trials—including patients with congenital heart disease, frail older adults, those with multimorbidity, and individuals from socioeconomically disadvantaged or rural backgrounds. Studies of adolescents and adults with congenital heart disease, for example, show that supervised rehabilitation is both feasible and safe in this population, improving exercise capacity and quality of life, yet referral remains the exception rather than the rule (Contributor 3).

A recent review further highlights how these "niche" populations often fall through the cracks of standard rehabilitation pathways, despite having much to gain from tailored interventions, flexible delivery models and closer integration with specialist care. Addressing their needs will require not only technical innovation, but also a shift in mindset: from a narrow, procedure-based view of eligibility towards a life-course, person-centred concept of cardiac rehabilitation as an adaptable framework for long-term cardiovascular health. Only then will the promise of rehabilitation extend to all those who could benefit from it—not just to the easiest patients to reach.

 https://doi.org/10.3390/jcm15041362

One of the most striking contributions in this issue is the report on a hybrid cardiac rehabilitation and symptom scoring programme for patients with inappropriate sinus tachycardia and postural orthostatic tachycardia syndrome referred for sinus node–sparing hybrid ablation (Contributor 4). These predominantly young women, often experiencing years of debilitating symptoms and diagnostic uncertainty, are almost invisible in traditional cardiac rehabilitation literature, yet here they are offered a structured, multidisciplinary pathway that combines early mobilisation, psychological support, respiratory therapy and home-based telerehabilitation. The high completion rates, marked reduction in Malmö POTS scores and favourable safety profile illustrate how thoughtfully designed rehabilitation can transform care even in highly specialised, previously neglected niches of cardiovascular medicine.

Another article in this issue focuses on women with heart failure, a group that is doubly disadvantaged: at higher risk of adverse outcomes, yet less likely to participate in cardiac rehabilitation (Contributor 5). The study highlights how traditional programmes often collide with the realities of women's daily lives—caregiving duties, household responsibilities and inflexible schedules—and how symptoms of anxiety, low mood or a tendency to prioritise others over themselves further reinforce avoidance or early dropout from rehabilitation. By documenting these gendered barriers in detail and linking them to concrete participation patterns, the authors remind us that improving access for women with heart failure will require not only medical optimisation, but also redesign of rehabilitation models that acknowledges their social roles, time constraints and psychological profiles.

Psychological factors are not a decorative add-on to cardiac rehabilitation; they are often the hidden engine that determines whether patients engage with, persevere in and ultimately benefit from the programme [7]. Recent work comparing different psychological interventions within multidisciplinary rehabilitation shows that targeted approaches such as individual counselling can meaningfully reduce anxiety and depression and improve illness perception, thereby creating the emotional and cognitive space needed for patients to change behaviour and adhere to long-term risk-factor management.

In contrast, studies examining clinical, anthropometric and lifestyle determinants of enrolment remind us that many decisions about rehabilitation are also shaped by more visible variables—age, comorbidities, symptom burden, obesity, smoking, as well as social factors such as distance to the centre or competing obligations. Patients with more severe heart failure, multiple coexisting conditions or lower functional capacity may be less frequently referred or may decline participation, while those with higher education and better baseline health literacy are more likely to enrol (Contributor 6). Bringing these psychological and clinical perspectives together underscores a simple truth: improving uptake of cardiac rehabilitation requires us to address both what patients feel and believe, and the structural realities that make joining a programme either feasible or impossible.

The picture would be incomplete without considering the role of family. A dedicated review from this Special Issue synthesises evidence showing that involving partners and relatives in cardiac rehabilitation can enhance communication with clinicians, improve patients' understanding of their condition and, in some studies, even reduce mortality and improve quality of life by strengthening emotional and practical support. At the same time, it cautions that overly intrusive involvement may threaten patients' sense of autonomy and privacy, underscoring the need for carefully negotiated boundaries so that family members become empowering allies rather than an additional source of pressure during recovery (Contributor 7).

Beyond formal psychological counselling, softer, often underestimated practices such as meditation and yoga are beginning to find their place alongside exercise and education in cardiac rehabilitation. In a recent pilot trial, adding transcendental meditation or yoga to

https://doi.org/10.3390/jcm15041362

standard post-surgical rehabilitation did not measurably alter retinal microcirculation, yet it underscored the feasibility of integrating such approaches into routine programmes and pointed towards their potential to reduce stress, modulate autonomic tone and support patients' overall sense of well-being (Contributor 8). When viewed together with broader data on mindfulness-based interventions in cardiovascular disease, these findings suggest that cultivating calm and attentional presence may be more than a pleasant extra—it may become a subtle but meaningful ally in helping patients sustain lifestyle change and cope with the long journey of recovery.

At the opposite end of the spectrum, another contribution in this issue descends to the cellular and subcellular consequences of exercise-based rehabilitation. By synthesising current knowledge on mitochondrial bioenergetics, this review links routine training prescriptions—frequency, intensity, interval structure—with mechanisms such as mitochondrial biogenesis, dynamics and mitophagy, arguing that at least part of the clinical benefit of rehabilitation is written into the way cardiomyocytes generate and recycle energy. In doing so, it offers a powerful reminder that when we prescribe a walking test or an interval session, we are not only improving peak oxygen uptake or six-minute walk distance, but also, quite literally, re-educating the heart at the level of its smallest power plants (Contributor 9).

Taken together, the works assembled in this Special Issue show cardiac rehabilitation in all its complexity: grounded in strong international guidelines, yet still underused; capable of adapting through digital and hybrid models; sensitive to gender, psychology and family dynamics; and reaching from social context down to mitochondrial function. Like the frog in the Brothers Grimm fairy tale, rehabilitation no longer needs to prove its royal lineage—the evidence is already there. What it now awaits is the collective "kiss" of implementation: clinicians who routinely refer, patients who are invited and supported to attend, policymakers who fund and prioritise programmes, and researchers who continue to refine and personalise interventions so that no group is left behind. When these elements finally come together, cardiac rehabilitation may at last shed its disguise and step fully into its rightful role as a central, visible, and irresistible part of modern cardiovascular care.

Conflicts of Interest: The authors declare no conflict of interest.

List of Contributions:

1. Bralewska, B.; Wykrota, J.; Kurpesa, M.; Kasprzak, J.D.; Cieślik-Guerra, U.; Wądołowska, E.; Rechciński, T. Cardiac Telerehabilitation After Acute Coronary Syndrome Ensures Similar Improvement in Exercise Capacity as Inpatient Rehabilitation, Regardless of the Age Profile of the Compared Groups. *J. Clin. Med.* **2025**, *14*, 3143. https://doi.org/10.3390/jcm14093143. PMID: 40364173; PMCID: PMC12072757.
2. Mori, E.; Ishii, H.; Matsuura, H.; Kono, Y.; Aoyagi, Y.; Shimizu, R.; Hiratsuka, T.; Sobue, Y.; Watanabe, E.; Kagaya, H. Effect of Introducing a Mini-Ergometer to the Ward Due to the COVID-19 Pandemic-Imposed Restrictions on Rehabilitation Centers on Physical Function: Cardiac Rehabilitation of Patients with Heart Failure. *J. Clin. Med.* **2025**, *14*, 5922. https://doi.org/10.3390/jcm14175922. PMID: 40943682; PMCID: PMC12429291.
3. Filipiak-Strzecka, D.; Bytyçi, I.; Bielecka-Dabrowa, A. How to Evaluate and Adjust the Recommended Level of Physical Activity in Patients with Congenital Heart Diseases? A Practical Approach. *J. Clin. Med.* **2025**, *14*, 8126. https://doi.org/10.3390/jcm14228126. PMID: 41303161; PMCID: PMC12653658.
4. Kornaszewska, M.; Wilczek-Banc, A.; Ratajska, A.; Piotrowicz, E.; Szkaradek, B.; Kowalewski, M.; Suwalski, P.; Ogorzelec, N.; Wileczek, A.; Zając, M.; et al. Implementation of a Hybrid Cardiac Rehabilitation and Symptom Scoring System in Patients with Inappropriate or Postural Sinus Tachycardia Referred for Sinus Node Sparing Hybrid Ablation. *J. Clin. Med.* **2025**, *14*, 5879. https://doi.org/10.3390/jcm14165879. PMID: 40869705; PMCID: PMC12387547.

5. Piotrowicz, E.; Główczyńska, R.; Szalewska, D.; Kowalik, I.; Orzechowski, P.; Pluta, S.; Kalarus, Z.; Mierzyńska, A.; Jaworska, I.; Irzmański, R.; et al. Effectiveness and Safety of Hybrid Comprehensive Telerehabilitation in Women with Heart Failure-A Subanalysis of the TELEREH-HF Randomized Clinical Trial. *J. Clin. Med.* **2026**, *15*, 694. https://doi.org/10.3390/jcm15020694. PMID: 41598632; PMCID: PMC12842170.
6. Kleinrok, A.; Krawczyk-Suszek, M.; Zams, B. The Impact of Selected Risk Factors on the Frequency of Cardiac Rehabilitation: Part I. *J. Clin. Med.* **2025**, *14*, 8289. https://doi.org/10.3390/jcm14238289. PMID: 41375592; PMCID: PMC12693505.
7. Popescu, G.; Maștaleru, A.; Oancea, A.; Costache, A.D.; Adam, C.A.; Rîpă, C.; Cumpăt, C.M.; Leon, M.M. Impact of Family Involvement in Cardiac Rehabilitation-Insights from a Literature Review. *J. Clin. Med.* **2025**, *14*, 6468. https://doi.org/10.3390/jcm14186468. PMID: 41010671; PMCID: PMC12471110.
8. Saloň, A.; Schmid-Zalaudek, K.; Steuber, B.; Rudlof, M.E.; Bartel, T.O.; Mächler, P.; Dorr, A.; Picha, R.; Fredriksen, P.M.; Nkeh-Chungag, B.N.; et al. Randomized Trial: A Pilot Study Investigating the Effects of Transcendental Meditation and Yoga Through Retinal Microcirculation in Cardiac Rehabilitation. *J. Clin. Med.* **2025**, *14*, 232. https://doi.org/10.3390/jcm14010232. PMID: 39797312; PMCID: PMC11722355.
9. Dziedzic, A.; Marek, K.; Niebrzydowski, P.; Szalewska, D.; Nowak, P.; Miller, E. Mitochondrial Bioenergetics and Cardiac Rehabilitation: Bridging Basic Science and Clinical Practice. *J. Clin. Med.* **2025**, *14*, 3949. https://doi.org/10.3390/jcm14113949. PMID: 40507710; PMCID: PMC12156409.

References

1. Visseren, F.L.J.; Mach, F.; Smulders, Y.M.; Carballo, D.; Koskinas, K.C.; Bäck, M.; Benetos, A.; Biffi, A.; Boavida, J.M.; Capodanno, D.; et al. 2021 ESC Guidelines on cardiovascular disease prevention in clinical practice. *Eur. J. Prev. Cardiol.* **2022**, *29*, 5–115. [CrossRef] [PubMed]
2. JCS Joint Working Group. Guidelines for Secondary Prevention of Myocardial Infarction (JCS 2011). *Circ. J.* **2013**, *77*, 231–248. [CrossRef] [PubMed]
3. Kotseva, K.; De Bacquer, D.; Jennings, C.; McEvoy, J.W.; Ryden, L.; Ray, K.K.; Lip, G.Y.H.; Erlund, I.; Ganly, S.; Vihervaara, T.; et al. Cardiac Rehabilitation in Patients with Coronary Heart Disease—Provision, Attendance, and Outcomes: Results from the INTERASPIRE Survey from Fourteen Countries Across Six WHO Regions. *Glob. Heart* **2025**, *20*, 75. [CrossRef] [PubMed] [PubMed Central]
4. Zhang, S.M.; Wu, Y.F.; Li, Z.Z.; Wang, C.S.; Wang, Y.; Xiao, N.; Du, H.Y.; Lin, S.; Du, M.Z.; Wu, Y.; et al. The Current Status of Cardiac Rehabilitation in China: A Cross-sectional National Survey. *Arch. Phys. Med. Rehabil.* **2026**, *Epub ahead of print*. [CrossRef] [PubMed]
5. Medina-Inojosa, J.R.; Chacin Suarez, A.S.; Murtala, A.B.; Hicks, J.B.; Harris, K.; Bennett, J.; Sperling, L.S. COVID-19 Pandemic: Wake-up Call and Accelerator for Cardiac Rehabilitation. *Can. J. Cardiol.* **2025**, *41*, S75–S85. [CrossRef] [PubMed]
6. Bäck, M.; Leosdottir, M.; Ekström, M.; Hambraeus, K.; Ravn-Fischer, A.; Borg, S.; Brosved, M.; Flink, M.; Hedin, K.; Lans, C.; et al. Feasibility, safety and patient perceptions of exercise-based cardiac telerehabilitation in a multicentre real-world setting after myocardial infarction-the remote exercise SWEDEHEART study. *Eur. Heart J. Digit. Health* **2025**, *6*, 508–518. [CrossRef] [PubMed] [PubMed Central]
7. Adachi, T.; Tsunekawa, Y.; Matsuoka, A.; Tanimura, D. Association between Big Five Personality Traits and Participation in Cardiac Rehabilitation in Japanese Patients with Cardiovascular Disease: A Retrospective Cohort Study. *Int. J. Environ. Res. Public Health* **2021**, *18*, 8589. [CrossRef] [PubMed] [PubMed Central]

 https://doi.org/10.3390/jcm15041362

Journal of
Clinical Medicine

MDPI

Article

Cardiac Telerehabilitation After Acute Coronary Syndrome Ensures Similar Improvement in Exercise Capacity as Inpatient Rehabilitation, Regardless of the Age Profile of the Compared Groups

Barbara Bralewska [1], Julia Wykrota [1], Małgorzata Kurpesa [2], Jarosław D. Kasprzak [2], Urszula Cieślik-Guerra [3], Ewa Wądołowska [3] and Tomasz Rechciński [2,*]

[1] Student Scientific Association, Medical University of Lodz, 90-419 Lodz, Poland; barbara.bralewska@student.umed.lodz.pl (B.B.); julia.wykrota@student.umed.lodz.pl (J.W.)
[2] 1st Department of Cardiology, Medical University of Lodz, 90-419 Lodz, Poland; malgorzata.kurpesa@umed.lodz.pl (M.K.); jaroslaw.kasprzak@umed.lodz.pl (J.D.K.)
[3] Department of Cardiac Rehabilitation, The Bieganski Hospital, 91-347 Lodz, Poland; cieursz@gmail.com (U.C.-G.)
* Correspondence: tomasz.rechcinski@office365.umed.pl

Abstract: Introduction: During the COVID-19 pandemic, the availability of cardiac rehabilitation (CR) was limited. On the other hand, during that period of epidemic restrictions, patients with acute coronary syndrome (ACS) required careful control and monitoring after coronary events. The aim of this study was to assess whether CR conducted during the epidemic restrictions in a remote mode ensured similar improvement in physical performance as CR conducted in a centre-based mode before the COVID-19 pandemic. **Material and Methods**: In this one-centre study, we compared the demographic and clinical profiles of patients after ACS who completed inpatient CR before the COVID-19 era with those of patients who completed telerehabilitation during the COVID-19 pandemic. We assessed the workload on the initial and final exercise tests (ExT) obtained by patients and compared the values of the differences between the final and initial ExT. The study included 359 patients (pts) participating in inpatient CR before October 2020 (the suspension of centre-based CR) and 60 pts who took part in telerehabilitation after July 2021 (the introduction of the tele-CR programme). Both inpatient and tele-CR were performed according to the guidelines of the Working Group for Cardiac Rehabilitation of the National Cardiac Society. A telemedic platform was used to control ECG, blood pressure and body mass of the pts participating in telerehabilitation. **Results**: The improvement of physical performance did not differ significantly between the two groups. The pts who completed telerehabilitation were significantly older than those who completed inpatient CR. The values of other parameters, such as the percentage of females, BMI, the percentage of pts with arterial hypertension and type 2 diabetes mellitus, as well as left ventricular ejection fraction did not differ significantly between the compared groups. Nor did the results of initial ExT expressed in METs, the results of final ExT and the improvement of workload understood as the difference between the final and initial results of ExT differ significantly—they were 7.7 ± 3.06 vs. 7.89 ± 2.98 with $p = 0.82$; 9.08 ± 0.29 vs. 8.98 ± 3.48 with $p = 0.84$, and 1 [0–2.2] vs. 1.2 [0–1.8] with $p = 0.17$, respectively. **Conclusions**: In our centre, telerehabilitation after acute coronary syndrome guaranteed an equally good improvement in physical capacity as that observed in inpatient CR patients, regardless of the difference in the age profile of the compared groups. These results encourage the popularization of telerehabilitation with remote monitoring of ECG, blood pressure and body mass.

Keywords: cardiac rehabilitation; COVID-19; telerehabilitation

1. Introduction

According to the guidelines of the European Society of Cardiology (ESC), comprehensive cardiac rehabilitation (CR) is classified as class IA as a method of treating patients after myocardial infarction, after myocardial revascularization, with chronic coronary syndrome, and with heart failure. In Poland, until 12 December 2015, telemedicine functioned rather as a theoretical concept, without any real possibility of its application. It was not until the Act of the 9th of October 2015 on the change of the Act on the Healthcare Information System and of certain other Acts (Journal of Laws, item 1991) and the amendment of the Act on the Medical and Dental Professions in December 2015 that its practical application was possible. One of the factors which had a major impact on the rapid development of cardiac telerehabilitation was the COVID-19 pandemic, when the availability of inpatient cardiac rehabilitation (CR) was completely abolished, and patients immediately after acute coronary syndromes (ACS) required careful monitoring and provision of rehabilitation opportunities.

The aim of this study was to assess whether remote cardiac rehabilitation conducted during the epidemic period (the study group) provided a similar improvement in exercise capacity as inpatient rehabilitation before the COVID-19 pandemic (the reference group).

2. Materials and Methods

In this retrospective study, we analysed data from 60 patients in the study group, who participated in cardiac telerehabilitation between 30 July 2021 and 30 June 2022. The total number of patients who participated in telerehabilitation was 98; those who were rehabilitated for reasons other than acute coronary syndrome, e.g., after valve replacement, electrotherapy, congestive heart failure, or Bentall surgery, were excluded. The final number of patients who participated in the study was 60. Among the women in the study group, one (9%) was professionally active, while the remaining 10 (91%) were retired. Among the men, 15 (31%) were professionally active and 34 (69%) were retired. In the reference group were 359 patients who participated in inpatient rehabilitation in the years preceding the pandemic at a tertiary referral centre. The patients in the study group and in the reference group were referred for rehabilitation after ACS and percutaneous coronary angioplasty or coronary artery bypass grafting.

In accordance with the requirements of the insurer (the National Health Fund), the telerehabilitation programme [1] took place during 24 sessions within a maximum of 90 consecutive days. Our centre preferred the patients to have rehabilitation sessions without breaks other than days off from work, but if necessary, the patient could take breaks between sessions. On the first day of the programme, the patient was admitted to the centre and qualified for the rehabilitation programme by a cardiologist. This qualification consisted of conducting an interview with the patient; a physical examination; determining their pharmacological treatment and its compliance with ESC standards (the percentages of patients from the study group taking various medications are presented in Table 1); analysis of the laboratory tests performed so far; measuring the patient's blood pressure, heart rate, body mass and height; and also an assessment of the patient's mental state by a psychologist. Patients were also checked for any contraindications to rehabilitation, such as anaemia with haemoglobin concentration below 10 g/l, inflammation, unstable angina pectoris, myocarditis, pulmonary embolism, peripheral embolism, heart failure in the period of decompensation or atrioventricular conduction disorders requiring the implantation of a cardiac pacemaker.

Table 1. Percentage comparison of the medications taken by patients in the study group.

Class of Medications	The Percentage (%) of Patients Taking the Medications
Statins	97
Beta blockers	94
Angiotensin-converting enzyme II inhibitors	90
Acetylsalicylic acid	85
Proton pump inhibitor (pantoprazole)	77
P2Y12 inhibitors	74
Calcium channel antagonists	22
Aldosterone receptor antagonists	18.3
Ezetimibe	18.3
Flozins	18.3
Trimetazidine	15
Thiazide diuretics	15
Ivabradine	10
Sartans	8.3

On the second day of the programme, the physician qualifying the patient for telerehabilitation performed an electrocardiographic stress test (ECG) according to the Bruce-Ramp protocol, assessed their heart rhythm, heart rate limit, and checked for the presence of electrocardiographic signs of myocardial ischemia or new disturbances of rhythm or conduction.

On days 3, 4, and 5 of the programme, patients from the study group were educated on how to use the telerehabilitation device. This included learning how to use the telerehabilitation monitoring equipment: measuring heart rate, blood pressure, body mass, following the planned exercise programme, and assessing their level of exertion according to the Borg scale. The patients also took part in meetings with a psychologist, who helped them to cope with possible symptoms of depression and anxiety related to the disease, and with a dietitian, who taught them the principles of preparing a healthy diet. On days 6–23, the actual rehabilitation of the patients took place. The training protocol was standardised for all patients. The training consisted of marching under heart rate control (the patients were advised to reach a training heart rate limit). Before each training session, during a telephone conversation, the patients answered questions about their current health, well-being, and medications taken. Then, they sent their resting ECG record as well as their blood pressure and body mass measurements to the monitoring centre—the doctor also had all previous measurements in the form of a graph (see Figure 1). The resting ECG was sent to the centre twice before the start of training, and then at 20 min intervals and after the training. In the transmitted ECG, it was possible to assess heart rhythm: whether it was sinus rhythm or not, whether there were arrhythmias (e.g., atrial fibrillation, premature ventricular or supraventricular extrasystoles). The system also allowed the measurement of the duration of the PQ interval, of the QT interval and of the QRS complex (Figure 2). If there were no contraindications, the patient received consent to start the training session. The telerehabilitation ECG was monitored several times during each session. For stationary patients, ECG was performed during the first three days of the programme and then only in the case of emerging complaints (palpitations, retrosternal pain). In order to improve exercise capacity, three forms of exercise were recommended: endurance training, respiratory muscle training, and resistance and stretching training. On the last day, a final exercise ECG test was performed according to the Bruce–Ramp protocol.

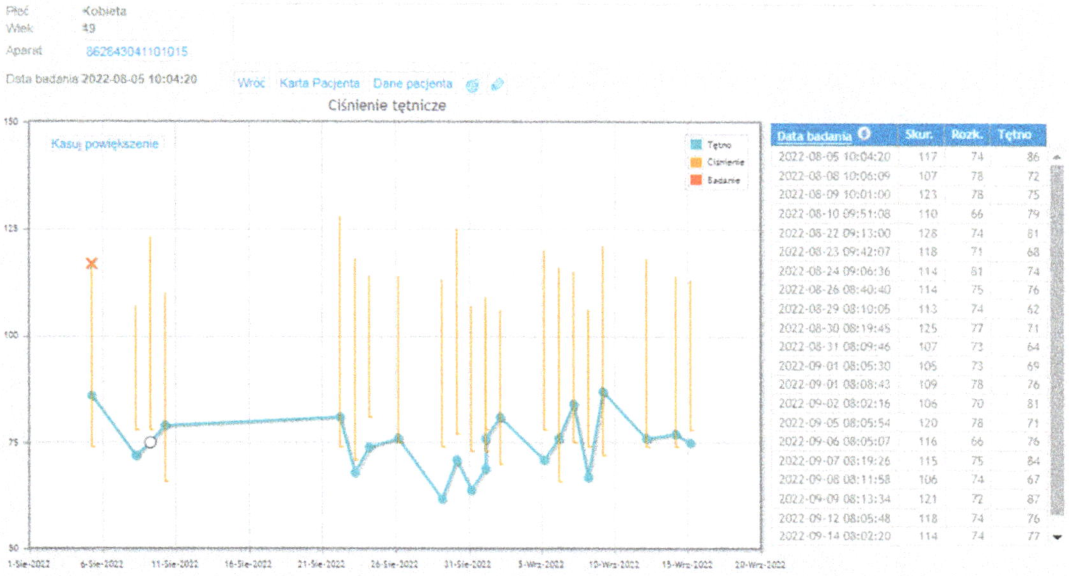

Figure 1. An example of a graph showing the blood pressure and the heart rate of a patient participating in telerehabilitation.

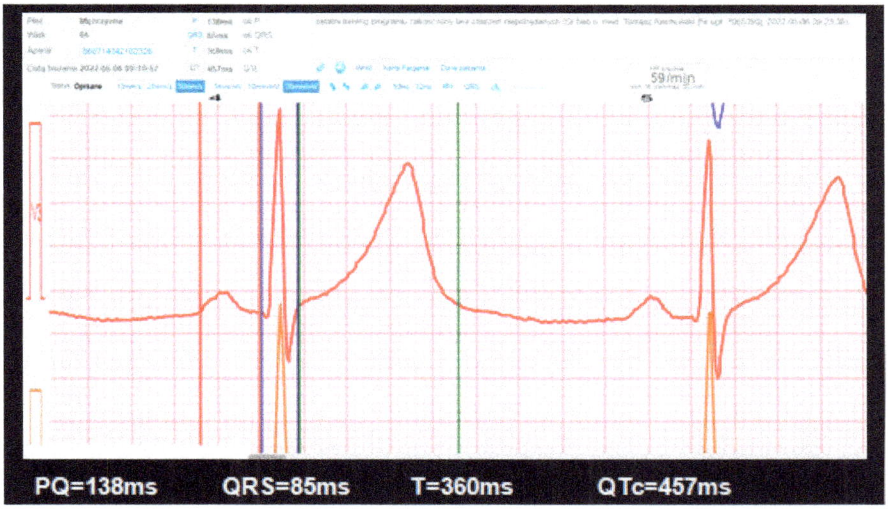

Figure 2. An example of measurement of the duration of the PQ interval (between red and purple lines), the QT interval (between purple and green lines) and the QRS complex (between purple and blue line).

Having been educated in the use of the telerehabilitation device, the patients performed training outside the centre; this included walking, cycling, and training on a stationary cycloergometer or treadmill (if available). If the training went according to plan, immediately after the training session, the telerehabilitation device, following a signal from the patient, sent an ECG to the monitoring centre via a mobile phone network. All the data sent by the patient were collected, analysed and stored in the monitoring centre in order to assess the safety, effectiveness and correctness of the rehabilitation carried out by the patients. On the basis of the assessment of the intensity of the exertion as perceived by the patients according to the Borg scale and of the electrocardiograms recorded during the training, decisions were made about the further rehabilitation process, and especially about the possibility or necessity of increasing or decreasing the load.

For patients from the reference group, training at the inpatient centre included morning gymnastics, endurance training on a cycloergometer (twice a day for 10–20 min), resistance training on a multi-gym, a rowing machine or an elliptical bike, Nordic walking and breathing training. The patients had also specially organized meetings with a psychologist, who conducted relaxation therapy, and with a dietitian, who analysed individual eating habits and recommended dietary modifications if necessary.

Both cardiac telerehabilitation and inpatient rehabilitation were conducted in accordance with the guidelines of the Working Group on Cardiac Rehabilitation of the Polish Cardiac Society. The electrocardiogram, blood pressure and body mass of patients participating in the remote rehabilitation program were monitored by means of the telemedicine platform manufactured by Pro-PLUS S.A. Polska.

Statistical analysis included the Mann–Whitney U test, Student's *t*-test and chi-square test.

3. Results

Patients from both groups were compared in terms of demographic and anthropomorphic as well as clinical characteristics, and exercise test results. The results are presented in Tables 2 and 3.

Table 2. A comparison of the demographic, anthropomorphic, and clinical characteristics of patients.

Demographic and Anthropomorphic Characteristics of Patients				
Variable	**The Study Group (Telerehabilitation)**	**The Reference Group (Inpatient CR)**	**Significance**	**All Rehabilitation Patients Participating in the Study**
Number of patients	60	359	-	419
Age [years]	63.7 ± 10.8	60.15 ± 9.8	0.003	60.66 ± 10
Females; number [%]	11, [18.3]	99, [27.5]	0.64	114, [27.2]
BMI	29.41 ± 4.65	28.0 ± 4.5	0.14	28.55 ± 4.5
Clinical characteristics				
Arterial hypertension; number [%]	40, [66.6]	255, [71.03]	0.49	295, [70.41]
Diabetes mellitus, number [%]	15, [25.0]	84, [23.39]	0.79	99, [23.63]
Left ventricular ejection fraction [%] mean ± SD	46.95 ± 8.16	47.48 ± 9.03	0.47	47.41 ± 8.91

Table 3. A comparison of the results of exercise tests of the patients participating in the study.

A Comparison of Physical Performance Between the Two Groups				
Variable	**The Study Group (Telerehabilitation)**	**The Reference Group (Inpatient CR)**	**Significance**	**All Rehabilitation Patients Participating in the Study**
Initial exercise test [MET]	7.89 ± 2.98	7.72 ± 3.06	0.82	7.75 ± 3.1
Final exercise test [MET]	8.98 ± 3.48	9.03 ± 3.29	0.84	9.03 ± 3.3
Improvement in workload capacity [MET] median [25–75%]	1.2 [0–1.8]	1.0 [0–2.2]	0.17	1.0 [0–2.2]

Statistical analysis showed a statistically significant difference only in the age of patients participating in the study in comparison with the reference group. The median age for the group of centre-based patients was 60.15, and for the patients participating in telerehabilitation it was 63.7.

There was also a numerical difference between the percentage of women in the study group and in the reference group, but (like the difference in mean BMI values) it turned out to be statistically not significant. Pearson's linear correlation coefficient between age and the final outcome of the exercise test was $r = -0.048$ with a determination coefficient of $R^2 = 0.002$, whereas the correlation between BMI and the final outcome of the exercise test was $r = -0.329$ and $R^2 = 0.108$. Weight control was mainly aimed at assessing fluid retention in patients taking diuretics. In the group monitored during the pandemic, we did not observe the need to change the dose of diuretics. None of the patients participating in the telerehabilitation were taking loop diuretics.

The result of the comparison of the increase in exercise capacity expressed in METs in the final exercise test as compared to the initial test and a comparison of these differences between the groups of patients from the centre-based group and those participating in telerehabilitation indicate no significant differences, as presented in Figure 3.

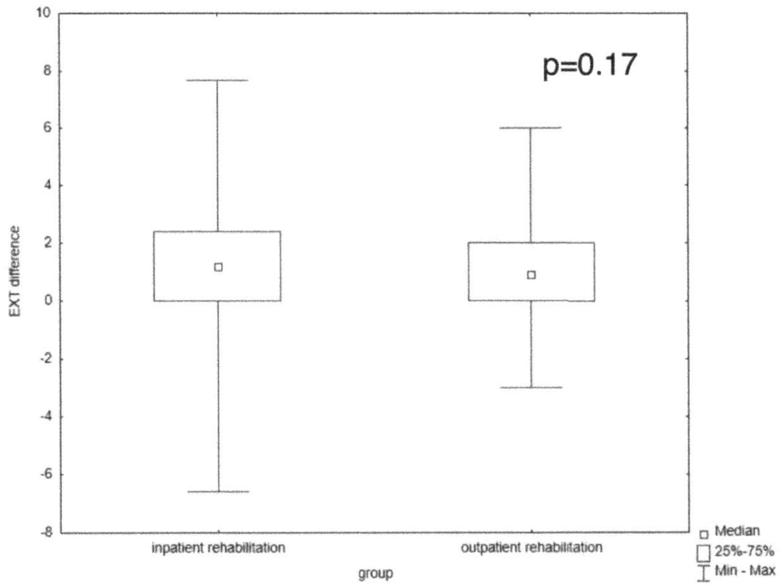

Figure 3. A comparison of patients from the inpatient rehabilitation group and patients participating in telerehabilitation in terms of increased exercise capacity. Y—the difference between the exercise capacity in the final exercise test and the result in the initial exercise test.

During the telerehabilitation of patients from the study group, adverse events occurred, presented in Table 4. However, they did not ultimately affect the deterioration of the final results of rehabilitation in terms of exercise capacity. They did not require interruption of the rehabilitation process and they disappeared when the pharmacotherapy used was modified or when new drugs were introduced [2].

Table 4. The percentage of adverse events in patients from the study group.

Adverse Events in Patients from the Study Group	The Percentage of Occurrence (%)
Suboptimal results of arterial blood pressure measurements	16.7
Bradycardia	6.7
A worsening of heart failure symptoms	5.1
Resting heart rate >75/min	3.3
Urinary tract infections	1.7
Episodes of atrial fibrillation	1.7

4. Discussion

The most important result of our work has been to show that there is no statistically significant difference in the improvement in exercise capacity between the group of patients participating in cardiac telerehabilitation and the group of patients participating in inpatient rehabilitation at the centre as assessed by an electrocardiographic exercise test performed according to the Bruce–Ramp protocol. This study also answers the question often asked by patients before they start cardiac telerehabilitation, which is this: what will be the probable result of the improvement in exercise capacity after the completion of the rehabilitation programme, and will it be similar to what they would obtain by participating in inpatient cardiac rehabilitation?

A statistically significant difference in age was found between the study group and the reference group. To determine if it could have any impact on the results, further research in this area would be needed. Another limitation of our study is the lack of information about digital literacy of patients participating in telerehabilitation.

Studies conducted to date indicate that during cardiac rehabilitation, patients improve their exercise capacity by an average of 1.5 METs [3]. Uznańska-Loch et al. [4] showed in their study that the highest probability of achieving the maximum improvement in exercise tolerance after cardiac rehabilitation is associated with the co-occurrence of left ventricular ejection fraction of >43% and a result of $\leq$8.4 METs in the initial exercise test. Age, BMI or sex were not significantly associated with the degree of improvement in exercise tolerance. Significant differences in the results occur in patients with normal and with reduced ejection fractions [5]. Heart failure with reduced left ventricular ejection fraction is a strong predictor of mortality after ACS on admission. Differences in the results achieved during cardiac rehabilitation are also related to gender [6]. Women achieve less improvement during cardiac rehabilitation, which can be explained by the higher age of the female population with ACS and with worse clinical results upon admission to the rehabilitation programme. The conclusion from the study by Bielecka-Dąbrowa et al. (the aim of which was to implement a health care model for patients with heart failure (HF) and to assess clinical and psychosocial differences between women and men in the study population) provides information that women suffer from HF symptoms more often and have a worse quality of life as assessed by the EQ-5D-5L than men, despite a better left ventricular ejection fraction [7].

Most studies conducted by other centres provide results similar to ours—cardiac telerehabilitation brings comparable results to centre-based cardiac rehabilitation in terms of exercise capacity and quality of life.

The study by Piotrowicz et al. [8], conducted, however, before the pandemic, included 152 patients with heart failure, mean age 58.1 $\pm$ 10.2 years, NYHA class II and III, and left ventricular ejection fraction $\leq$40%. The patients were randomly assigned to either home-based cardiac rehabilitation with ECG telemonitoring (n = 77) or conventional outpatient cardiac rehabilitation (n = 75). All the participants completed an eight-week cardiac rehabilitation programme. The two groups were comparable in terms of demographic and clinical characteristics, as well as pharmacological treatment. The efficacy of cardiac rehabilitation was evaluated on the basis of changes in the New York Heart Association (NYHA) functional class, in peak oxygen uptake (VO_2 peak) during cardiopulmonary exercise testing, in the distance achieved in the 6-min walk test, and in the scores from the SF-36 quality of life questionnaire. Significant improvements were observed in all the parameters assessed in both the standard rehabilitation group and the telerehabilitation group.

Further evidence supporting the efficacy of telerehabilitation is provided by the study conducted by Avila et al. [9], in which 90 patients with coronary artery disease (including 80 men) were randomly allocated in a 1:1:1 ratio to three groups: home-based rehabilitation (n = 30), centre-based rehabilitation (n = 30), and a control group receiving no rehabilitation (n = 30). The findings demonstrated that home-based exercise rehabilitation was as effective as the traditional, supervised centre-based programme. Importantly, no significant differences were observed between these two intervention groups in terms of final exercise capacity or physical activity levels.

In a separate study, Bernocchi et al. [10] investigated the feasibility and effectiveness of a four-month integrated home-based telerehabilitation programme (Telereab-HBP) in patients diagnosed with chronic obstructive pulmonary disease (COPD) and coexisting chronic heart failure (CHF). The primary outcome measure was the distance covered in the six-minute walk test (6MWT), while secondary outcomes included time to clinical events (hospitalization and mortality), the severity of dyspnoea, exercise activity levels, functional disability, and health-related quality of life. The Telereab-HBP intervention comprised a remote monitoring of cardiorespiratory parameters, weekly nurse-led telephone consultations, and a structured exercise regimen supervised weekly by a physiotherapist. Outcomes were reassessed following a two-month, non-interventional follow-up period. A total of 112 patients were randomised evenly between the intervention and the control groups (n = 56 per group), with a mean age ± standard deviation of 70 ± 9 years; 82.1% of participants were male. Interestingly, a comparable gender distribution was observed in our study, with 82% of participants in the telerehabilitation group and 72% in the inpatient rehabilitation group being male. The findings reported by Bernocchi et al. demonstrated a significant improvement in the 6MWT distance following the four-month programme, leading to the conclusion that this approach—combining remote physiological monitoring and regular professional consultations—is both feasible and efficacious in elderly patients with concurrent COPD and CHF.

In the study by Kraal et al. [11], 90 patients at a low or moderate cardiovascular risk, who were starting cardiac rehabilitation, were randomised to 3 months of home-based training with telemonitoring advice or to in-centre training. Physical fitness improved significantly at discharge and at one-year follow-up ($p < 0.01$) in both groups, with no significant differences between the two groups. The levels of exercise activity did not change significantly during the one-year follow-up. The health care costs were numerically lower in the "home" group, but this difference was not statistically significant. The authors of that study reached similar conclusions to the ones that we present in our article: telerehabilitation yielded equally good results as in-hospital cardiac rehabilitation. Although adherence to the training recommendations was similar in both groups, satisfaction with the rehabilitation programme was higher in the home-based group. Although in our study we did not conduct a survey on the degree of satisfaction with the form of rehabilitation, no patient reported any problems with operating the telerehabilitation equipment or barriers related to this form of training.

In the randomised study conducted by Bravo-Escobar et al. [12], 28 patients with stable coronary artery disease and moderate cardiovascular risk were enrolled. Fourteen patients were assigned to a conventional hospital-based cardiac rehabilitation program (the control group), while the remaining 14 participated in a home-based program with mixed supervision (the intervention group). The average BMI and mean age of the participants were comparable to those observed in our study. Notably, as in our cohort, the home-based group had a slightly higher mean age than the hospital-based group. No significant differences were observed between the two groups regarding exercise duration, METs achieved during the stress test, or the 1-min recovery index—all of which improved in both groups following the rehabilitation programme.

An interesting modern method for monitoring the course of telerehabilitation is the use of smartwatches by patients described by Mitropoulos et al. [13]. A randomised trial was designed to assess the effects of real-time monitoring of cardiac telerehabilitation using smartwatches in people who had recently had a myocardial infarction. All the patients completed baseline and follow-up measurements after 24 weeks, which assessed peak oxygen uptake, the mean daily step count, distance, and calories. The online group showed similar improvements in the mean daily step count and the mean daily walking distance after 24 weeks as the gym-based exercise group. There were no adverse events related to exercise during the study. The results of the study indicate that a real-time supervised exercise programme of cardiac rehabilitation using smartwatch technology to monitor the haemodynamic response in patients with coronary artery disease and after a myocardial infarction is as effective as the gym-based exercise programme.

Researchers also compared the effectiveness of outpatient hospital-based cardiac rehabilitation and telerehabilitation in patients after coronary artery bypass grafting (CABG) surgery [14]. Similarly to our study, the mean age of patients in the "home group" was slightly higher than the mean age of patients in the "hospital group". Measurements encompassed incremental shuttle walk test (ISWT) performance, psychosocial questionnaire scores, and body composition, measured at baseline, at the end of the eight-week intervention, and again at the end of a four-week post-intervention follow-up. Both the home-based and hospital-based cardiac rehabilitation groups demonstrated improvements in ISWT duration compared to baseline values. Home-based rehabilitation proved to be equally effective as traditional outpatient rehabilitation in enhancing exercise capacity among post-coronary artery bypass grafting patients. Furthermore, the home-based approach appeared to be superior in sustaining these gains over the follow-up period.

Interesting results are presented in the study by Gu et al. [15]. They analysed a cohort of stable patients with coronary artery disease (CAD) who had undergone percutaneous coronary angioplasty and who participated in two different modes of the cardiac rehabilitation programme after being discharged from hospital. CR took place in two periods: from January 2019 to December 2019 (inpatient CR) and from May 2020 to May 2021 (remote CR). Exercise capacity was assessed using the 6 min walk test (6MWT), oxygen uptake at peak exercise (VO2max), and anaerobic respiratory threshold (VO2AT) before discharge, after 8 weeks of CR and after 12 weeks of CR, performed either in the centre or remotely at home. No adverse events occurred during the programme. Patients from both groups increased their walking distance in the 6MWT test with higher VO2max after 8 and 12 weeks. The patients participating in telerehabilitation showed better results in terms of anxiety and depression levels in comparison with the patients from inpatient rehabilitation.

Other cardiology studies on telemedicine raise important and interesting issues. The aim of a prospective study of Mariani et al. [16] was to analyse the feasibility and effectiveness of virtual visits compared to traditional in-person visits and to evaluate the experience of patients receiving remote care in clinical electrophysiology. The study focused on the following indicators: (1) improvement in complaints after the initial visit, (2) resolution of remote monitoring (RM) alerts during the follow-up, (3) need for emergency hospitalisation and (4) patient satisfaction as assessed using the Patient Satisfaction Questionnaire-18 (PSQ-18). Compared with in-person visits, virtual visits produced comparable results in terms of reduction of the number of RM alerts and of the frequency of symptoms at follow-up, with no differences in terms of urgent hospitalisation. Furthermore, patients rated virtual visits as more satisfactory than in-person visits. These results confirm that remote care is not only feasible, but also as effective as traditional care, with high levels of patient satisfaction.

The aim of the study of Ankışhan [17] was to develop new speech signal features to capture the relationship between voice recordings and blood pressure (BP). In this context, the literature describes a database containing the vowels/a/, recorded at different blood pressure values, under controlled environmental and room conditions. Tools such as convolutional neural networks for regression (CNN-R), support vector machines for regression (SVM-R) and multilinear regression (MLR) were used to predict BP values on the basis of extracted features. The experiments showed that the highest accuracy in predicting systolic BP values was achieved using CNN-R for the vowels/a/. The results obtained suggest that the proposed feature vector (FVx) reflects the relationship between blood pressure and vocal traits, opening up the possibility of using it in patient BP monitoring systems.

The limitation of our work is the small size of the study group, but this group comes from a unique period during the COVID-19 pandemic, when the only form of cardiac rehabilitation for patients after a myocardial infarction was telerehabilitation. Gathering a similar group of patients in the current period—outside the period of restrictions related to the pandemic—would be impossible owing to the fact that currently, patients and doctors have a choice between three forms of cardiac rehabilitation—inpatient rehabilitation, outpatient rehabilitation in the centre, and telerehabilitation (outside the centre).

5. Conclusions

In our centre, telerehabilitation after acute coronary syndrome performed during the COVID-19 pandemic guaranteed an equally good improvement in exercise capacity as that observed in patients undergoing inpatient rehabilitation, regardless of the difference in the age profile of the compared groups. These results, compared with studies from different centres and from different periods, encourage the popularization of the mode of cardiac rehabilitation based on the remote monitoring of ECG, arterial blood pressure and body mass.

Author Contributions: Conceptualization, T.R. and B.B.; methodology, T.R.; software, J.W.; validation, J.W. and B.B.; formal analysis, T.R.; investigation, E.W.; resources, U.C.-G.; data curation, J.W.; writing—original draft preparation, B.B.; writing—review and editing, T.R.; visualization, B.B.; supervision, J.D.K.; project administration, M.K. All authors have read and agreed to the published version of the manuscript.

Funding: This research received no external funding.

Institutional Review Board Statement: Ethical review and approval were waived for this study due to its retrospective nature and the use of patient data for which consent is not required as in experimental studies. All patients signed informed consent about use of their anonymized data in that study.

Informed Consent Statement: Informed consent was obtained from all subjects involved in the study.

Data Availability Statement: The source data available from the corresponding author.

Acknowledgments: We thank Janusz Wróblewski, for his linguistic help with the manuscript.

Conflicts of Interest: The authors declare no conflicts of interest.

References

1. Jegier, A.; Szalewska, D.; Mawlichanów, A.; Bednarczyk, T.; Eysymontt, Z.; Gałaszek, M.; Mamcarz, A.; Mierzyńska, A.; Piotrowicz, E.; Piotrowicz, R.; et al. Comprehensive cardiac rehabilitation as the keystone in the secondary prevention of cardiovascular disease. *Kardiol. Pol.* **2021**, *79*, 901–916. [CrossRef] [PubMed]
2. Bralewska, B.; Wykrota, J.; Kurpesa, M.; Kasprzak, J.D.; Cieślik-Guerra, U.; Wądołowska, E.; Rechciński, T. Adverse events during a cardiac telerehabilitation program: A single-center study. *Kardiol. Pol.* **2024**, *82*, 886–888. [CrossRef] [PubMed]
3. Abu-Haniyeh, A.; Shah, N.P.; Wu, Y.; Cho, L.; Ahmed, H.M. Predictors of cardiorespiratory fitness improvement in phase II cardiac rehabilitation. *Clin. Cardiol.* **2018**, *41*, 1563–1569. [CrossRef] [PubMed]
4. Uznańska-Loch, B.; Wądołowska, E.; Wierzbowska-Drabik, K.; Cieślik-Guerra, U.; Kasprzak, J.D.; Kurpesa, M.; Rechciński, T. Left ventricular systolic function and initial exercise capacity—Their importance for results of cardiac rehabilitation after acute coronary syndrome. *Explor. Cardiol.* **2023**, *1*, 26–34. [CrossRef]
5. Brezinov, O.P.; Klempfner, R.; Zekry, S.B.; Goldenberg, I.; Kuperstein, R. Prognostic value of ejection fraction in patients admitted with acute coronary syndrome. *Medicine* **2017**, *96*, e6226. [CrossRef] [PubMed]
6. Feola, M.; Garnero, S.; Daniele, B.; Mento, C.; Dell'Aira, F.; Chizzolini, G.; Testa, M. Gender differences in the efficacy of cardiovascular rehabilitation in patients after cardiac surgery procedures. *PubMed* **2015**, *12*, 575–579. [CrossRef]
7. Bielecka-Dąbrowa, A.; Trzmielak, D.; Sakowicz, A.; Janikowski, K.; Banach, M. Gender differences in efficiency of the telemedicine care of heart failure patients. The results from the TeleEduCare-HF study. *Arch. Med. Sci.* **2024**, *20*, 1797–1808. [CrossRef] [PubMed]
8. Piotrowicz, E.; Baranowski, R.; Bilinska, M.; Stepnowska, M.; Piotrowska, M.; Wójcik, A.; Korewicki, J.; Chojnowska, L.; Malek, L.A.; Klopotowski, M.; et al. A new model of home-based telemonitored cardiac rehabilitation in patients with heart failure: Effectiveness, quality of life, and adherence. *Eur. J. Heart Fail.* **2010**, *12*, 164–171. [CrossRef] [PubMed]
9. Avila, A.; Claes, J.; Buys, R.; Azzawi, M.; Vanhees, L.; Cornelissen, V. Home-based exercise with telemonitoring guidance in patients with coronary artery disease: Does it improve long-term physical fitness? *Eur. J. Prev. Cardiol.* **2019**, *27*, 367–377. [CrossRef] [PubMed]
10. Bernocchi, P.; Vitacca, M.; La Rovere, M.T.; Volterrani, M.; Galli, T.; Baratti, D.; Paneroni, M.; Campolongo, G.; Sposato, B.; Scalvini, S. Home-based telerehabilitation in older patients with chronic obstructive pulmonary disease and heart failure: A randomised controlled trial. *Age Ageing* **2017**, *47*, 82–88. [CrossRef] [PubMed]
11. Kraal, J.J.; Van Den Akker-Van Marle, M.E.; Abu-Hanna, A.; Stut, W.; Peek, N.; Kemps, H.M. Clinical and cost-effectiveness of home-based cardiac rehabilitation compared to conventional, centre-based cardiac rehabilitation: Results of the FIT@Home study. *Eur. J. Prev. Cardiol.* **2017**, *24*, 1260–1273. [CrossRef] [PubMed]
12. Bravo-Escobar, R.; González-Represas, A.; Gómez-González, A.M.; Montiel-Trujillo, A.; Aguilar-Jimenez, R.; Carrasco-Ruíz, R.; Salinas-Sánchez, P. Effectiveness and safety of a home-based cardiac rehabilitation programme of mixed surveillance in patients with ischemic heart disease at moderate cardiovascular risk: A randomised, controlled clinical trial. *BMC Cardiovasc. Disord.* **2017**, *17*, 66. [CrossRef] [PubMed]
13. Mitropoulos, A.; Anifanti, M.; Koukouvou, G.; Ntovoli, A.; Alexandris, K.; Kouidi, E. Exploring the effects of real-time online cardiac telerehabilitation using wearable devices compared to gym-based cardiac exercise in people with a recent myocardial infarction: A randomised controlled trial. *Front. Cardiovasc. Med.* **2024**, *11*, 1410616. [CrossRef] [PubMed]
14. Taktoni, M.; Thow, M.T.M.; Seenan, C.S. A randomized controlled trial of an eight-week cardiac rehabilitation home verse hospital exercise programme for post coronary cardiac bypass patients. *Eur. Heart J.* **2024**, *45* (Suppl. 1), ehae666.1443. [CrossRef]
15. Gu, J.; Tong, X.; Meng, S.; Xu, S.; Huang, J. Remote cardiac rehabilitation program during the COVID-19 pandemic for patients with stable coronary artery disease after percutaneous coronary intervention: A prospective cohort study. *BMC Sports Sci. Med. Rehabil.* **2023**, *15*, 79. [CrossRef] [PubMed]
16. Mariani, M.V.; Pierucci, N.; Forleo, G.B.; Schiavone, M.; Bernardini, A.; Gasperetti, A.; Mitacchione, G.; Mei, M.; Giunta, G.; Piro, A.; et al. The Feasibility, Effectiveness and Acceptance of Virtual Visits as Compared to In-Person Visits among Clinical Electrophysiology Patients during the COVID-19 Pandemic. *J. Clin. Med.* **2023**, *12*, 620. [CrossRef] [PubMed]
17. Ankışhan, H. Blood pressure prediction from speech recordings. *Biomed. Signal Process. Control* **2020**, *58*, 101842. [CrossRef]

Journal of
Clinical Medicine

MDPI

Article

Effect of Introducing a Mini-Ergometer to the Ward Due to the COVID-19 Pandemic-Imposed Restrictions on Rehabilitation Centers on Physical Function: Cardiac Rehabilitation of Patients with Heart Failure

Etsuko Mori [1,*], Hideki Ishii [2], Hirotaka Matsuura [3], Yuji Kono [4], Yoichiro Aoyagi [3,5], Rio Shimizu [1], Tomoyasu Hiratsuka [1], Yoshihiro Sobue [6], Eiichi Watanabe [6] and Hitoshi Kagaya [3,7]

1. Department of Rehabilitation, Fujita Health University Bantane Hospital, Nagoya 454-8509, Aichi, Japan; rio970714@gmail.com (R.S.); hira@fujita-hu.ac.jp (T.H.)
2. Department of Cardiovascular Medicine, Graduate School of Medicine, Gunma University, Maebashi 371-8511, Gunma, Japan; hkishii@gunma-u.ac.jp
3. Department of Rehabilitation Medicine, School of Medicine, Fujita Health University, Toyoake 470-1192, Aichi, Japan; hero850411@yahoo.co.jp (H.M.); yyy@rc5.so-net.ne.jp (Y.A.); hkagaya2@ncgg.go.jp (H.K.)
4. Department of Rehabilitation, Fujita Health University Hospital, Toyoake 470-1192, Aichi, Japan; yt-kono@fujita-hu.ac.jp
5. Department of Rehabilitation Medicine, Graduate School of Medicine, Nippon Medical School, Tokyo 113-8602, Japan
6. Division of Cardiology, Department of Internal Medicine, Fujita Health University Bantane Hospital, Nagoya 454-8509, Aichi, Japan; sobue@fujita-hu.ac.jp (Y.S.); enwatan@fujita-hu.ac.jp (E.W.)
7. Department of Rehabilitation Medicine, National Center for Geriatrics and Gerontology, Obu 474-8511, Aichi, Japan

* Correspondence: m-etsuko@fujita-hu.ac.jp; Tel.: +81-52-321-8171

Abstract: Background/Objectives: The COVID-19 pandemic restrictions had negative effects on cardiac rehabilitation. The difference in the location of cardiac rehabilitation practice during the COVID-19 pandemic decreased the amount of aerobic exercise and the patient's physical function at discharge. Therefore, we introduced a mini-ergometer to the ward to provide quantitative aerobic exercise. This study aimed to evaluate physical function at discharge after the introduction of a mini-ergometer to the ward in patients with heart failure. **Methods**: We included a total of 117 consecutive patients who were admitted to a university hospital and underwent a cardiac rehabilitation program for heart failure between June 2020 and September 2022. Patients were divided into two groups: Group A (n = 54), which included those admitted before the introduction of the mini-ergometer, and Group B (n = 63), which included those admitted after the introduction of the mini-ergometer. Data, including age, sex, and functional status, were obtained. Additionally, the duration of each rehabilitation exercise was measured. **Results**: Group B had a significantly higher 6 min walking distance at discharge than Group A (Group A: 236.0 m vs. Group B: 290.0 m, $p = 0.020$). Furthermore, Group B had a significantly longer ergometer exercise duration than Group A (Group A: 0 min vs. Group B: 25.0 min, $p < 0.001$). **Conclusions**: The results showed that the introduction of the mini-ergometer to the ward could ensure quantitative exercise loads even under restricted access to rehabilitation centers during the COVID-19 outbreak, thereby improving physical function at discharge in patients with heart failure.

Keywords: cardiac rehabilitation; inpatient rehabilitation; physical performance; COVID-19; controlled training; ward rehabilitation; ergometer exercise; heart failure; rehabilitation unit

1. Introduction

Aerobic exercise during cardiac rehabilitation is strongly recommended for patients with cardiovascular diseases [1]. It is a cornerstone of exercise prescription and plays a crucial role in rehabilitation. Beneficial effects of aerobic exercise in patients with cardiovascular disease have been demonstrated, including (1) improvement in left ventricular ejection fraction (LVEF) [2], (2) reduction in hospital readmission rates [3], (3) enhancement of quality of life [3], (4) the advantage of improving exercise tolerance [3–5], (5) improving walking speed [6], and (6) enhancing muscle strength [7]. Aerobic exercise in cardiac rehabilitation programs is mainly performed using a bicycle ergometer or treadmill installed in rehabilitation centers [8].

The COVID-19 pandemic-imposed restrictions on cardiac rehabilitation [9–11]. Kida et al. [11] conducted a survey involving 37 cardiac rehabilitation facilities in Japan during the early stage of the COVID-19 pandemic and reported that 49% of the facilities had temporarily suspended group exercise rehabilitation. However, all facilities maintained individual inpatient cardiac rehabilitation [11]. The Japanese Association of Cardiac Rehabilitation recommends cardiac rehabilitation standard programs for conducting exercise therapy in the rehabilitation unit after the acute phase mobilization program [12]. However, cardiac rehabilitation programs were implemented mainly in wards instead of rehabilitation centers to avoid the "three Cs," including crowded places, close-contact settings, and confined and enclosed spaces [13]. In our previous study [14], the effect of modified rehabilitation therapy performed in wards was compared with that of conventional therapies performed in rehabilitation centers where exercise on a treadmill and cardiopulmonary exercise testing were available. Patients admitted during the COVID-19 outbreak showed a significantly shorter ergometer exercise time, lower 6 min walking distance (6MWD), and lower walking speed at discharge than those admitted before the COVID-19 outbreak [14]. The difference in the location of cardiac rehabilitation practice during the COVID-19 pandemic might have affected the rehabilitation modality and the patient's physical function at discharge. Therefore, a mini-ergometer was introduced to the ward to provide quantitative aerobic exercise, even under restricted access to rehabilitation centers. We hypothesized that the introduction of a mini-ergometer to the ward would lead to greater improvement in physical function at discharge. Therefore, this study aimed to compare physical function at discharge before and after the introduction of a mini-ergometer to the ward in patients with heart failure.

2. Materials and Methods

2.1. Patients

Emergency patients who were admitted to our hospitals between June 2020 and September 2022 due to worsening heart failure and underwent cardiac rehabilitation were enrolled in this study. The inclusion criteria were patients aged 18 years and those who could complete the 6MWD measurement at discharge. The exclusion criteria included those with a history of COVID-19 infection, those who were readmitted during the study period, those with severe dementia, those with a history of neuromuscular disease, and those who did not wish to participate. In order to exclude acute infection, COVID-19 testing was performed for all patients at the time of admission.

The patients were divided into two groups: those admitted before the introduction of the mini-ergometer (Group A, April 2020–June 2021) and those admitted after the introduction of the mini-ergometer (Group B, July 2021–September 2022). Based on previous reports, the expected difference in 6MWD between groups was approximately 80 m, and the estimated standard deviation was around 190 m, resulting in a Cohen's d of approximately 0.42 [14]. Under these conditions ($\alpha = 0.05$, power = 0.80), the required sample size is estimated to be between 110 and 120 participants. Therefore, the sample size was regarded as appropriate for the purposes of this study.

2.2. Study Design and Protocols

This was a retrospective observational study conducted using our single-center database. This study was conducted in accordance with the principles of the Declaration of Helsinki and approved by the Research Ethics Committee of the institution (Approval No.: HM20-538). Informed consent was obtained using the opt-out method approved by the Committee.

2.3. Data Collection

Patients' demographic and clinical characteristics were obtained from the medical records. During hospitalization, the patients' demographic and clinical characteristics were evaluated, including blood investigation, heart failure severity, cardiac function, physical function, cognitive function, activities of daily living (ADL), and cardiac rehabilitation program. Additionally, age, sex, systolic blood pressure at admission, body mass index, comorbidities, and medication were recorded as demographic characteristics. Each patient's serum hemoglobin, albumin, and sodium concentrations were obtained, and the glomerular filtration rate was estimated from the blood investigation results at admission. The geriatric nutritional risk index was calculated from individually obtained serum albumin levels and body weights as follows [15]: geriatric nutritional risk index = [14.89 × albumin (g/dL)] + [41.7 × (body weight/ideal body weight)]. These blood parameters were obtained from samples collected in the outpatient laboratory at the time of hospital admission.

2.4. Heart Failure Severity and Cardiac Function

Evaluation of HF severity was conducted using N-terminal pro-brain natriuretic peptide (NT-proBNP). Cardiac function was evaluated by LVEF, a parameter of the left ventricular systolic function obtained via echocardiography and New York Heart Association (NYHA) functional class. Echocardiographic assessments were performed by one medical technologist per patient. Upon completion of the assessment, the findings were reviewed and approved by a cardiologist.

2.5. Physical Function

Physical function was assessed 3 days before discharge using the 6MWD, grip strength, isometric knee extensor muscle strength (KEMS), walking speed, functional reach test, and waist circumference. Additionally, grip strength and walking speed were assessed at the start of cardiac rehabilitation. The 6MWD test was performed in accordance with the guidelines of the American Thoracic Society [16]. Grip strength was measured using a digital grip strength dynamometer (T.K.K.5401, Takei Scientific Instruments, Niigata, Japan). Patients exerted maximum effort twice with their left and right hands, with the upper limb lowered parallel to the trunk in the sitting position. The maximum value obtained was used in the analysis. The KEMS was measured using a digital handheld dynamometer (mTasF-1, Anima, Tokyo, Japan). Patients were instructed to remain in the sitting posture, and the dynamometer's sensor pad was attached to the distal part of the lower leg. The strap from the sensor pad was then attached horizontally to the leg of the platform to fix the hip and knee joints at 90°. Patients were asked to extend the knee joint twice on both sides to push the sensor, and the maximum value was recorded. The

KEMS was transformed into newtons adjusted by weight (N/kg). The walking speed was measured using the usual 10 m walk test. Patients were instructed to walk at their usual pace for 14 m, and the middle 10 m was timed. The test was completed twice, and the fastest speed was used in the analysis. The waist circumference was measured in the standing posture, at the height of the navel, and at the time of exhalation using a measuring tape. The functional reach test was measured as the length of the shortened rod after reaching forward as much as possible using the expandable rod [17]. The maximum circumference of the calf was measured with a measuring tape. The maximum calf circumference was measured while sitting without the feet touching the floor.

2.6. Cognitive Function and ADL Assessment

Cognitive function was assessed using the Mini-Mental State Examination-Japan (MMSE-J) 3 days before discharge. The MMSE-J comprises 11 categories, with a total score of 30 [18]. Cognitive function was assessed by a therapist in a quiet, private room. The ability of patients to perform ADLs was assessed using the Functional Independence Measure (FIM) [19] at admission and discharge. FIM included 13 motor and 5 cognitive items. Each item had a 7-point ordinal scale from total assistance (a score of 1) to complete independence (a score of 7). Additionally, the FIM gain (the difference between FIM score at discharge and FIM score at admission) and FIM efficiency (FIM gain divided by length of hospitalization) were assessed, which are commonly used to evaluate the degree of improvement.

2.7. Rehabilitation Program

The content and duration of the rehabilitation program, including assessment, range of motion exercise, sitting up exercise, sitting exercise, standing exercise, walking exercise, ergometer exercise, resistance training, ADL training, and other parameters recorded every 5 min, were evaluated. A fitness bicycle (Model CMMY-201901; QLEE, Guangzhou, China) was used as the mini-ergometer.

2.8. Exercise Training

All patients underwent general cardiac rehabilitation according to the Standard Cardiac Rehabilitation Program for Heart Failure [12]. Specifically, patients underwent rehabilitation in the ward until their general condition stabilized. If they were able to walk steadily, they subsequently received exercise therapy at the rehabilitation center. The study population included a large proportion of elderly individuals, and individualized programs, including training in essential daily living skills, were implemented as follows: Assessment, Range of motion exercise, Sitting up exercise, Sitting exercise, Standing exercise, Walking exercise, Ergometer exercise (Figure 1), Resistance training, and ADL training. Exercise intensity was individually determined, and the rehabilitation sessions were monitored using subjective ratings of perceived exertion based on the Borg scale. All patients underwent cardiac rehabilitation, consisting of 40-to-80 min sessions, five days a week during at admission.

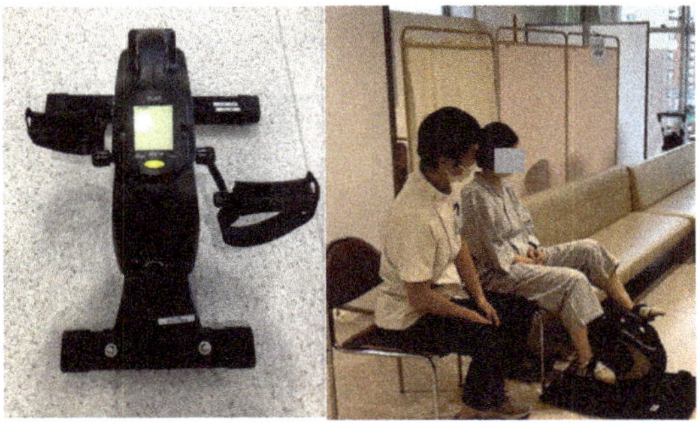

(**a**) (**b**)

Figure 1. Ergometer exercise. (**a**) The mini-ergometer employed in this study, (**b**) Exercise training with a mini-ergometer.

2.9. Statistical Analysis

Data were presented as median (interquartile range) for numerical variables and number (percentage) for categorical variables. In between-group comparisons, categorical variables were analyzed using the chi-square test, and numerical variables were analyzed using the Mann–Whitney U test. All analyses were performed using the SPSS 27.0 software package (SPSS Inc., Tokyo, Japan). A p-value < 0.05 was considered statistically significant.

3. Results

Among 164 patients, 47 were excluded from data analyses. Of the 117 included patients, 54 and 63 were categorized into groups A (range of age, 38–98 years) and B (range of age, 47–98 years), respectively (Figure 2). The demographic data of the patients at admission are presented in Table 1. Group B showed a lower walking speed than Group A at the start of cardiac rehabilitation (Group A: 0.9 m/s vs. Group B: 0.7 m/s, $p = 0.065$). No significant difference in the duration of the cardiac rehabilitation program provided in the ward was observed between the two groups (Group A: 720.0 min vs. Group B: 660.0 min, $p = 0.109$).

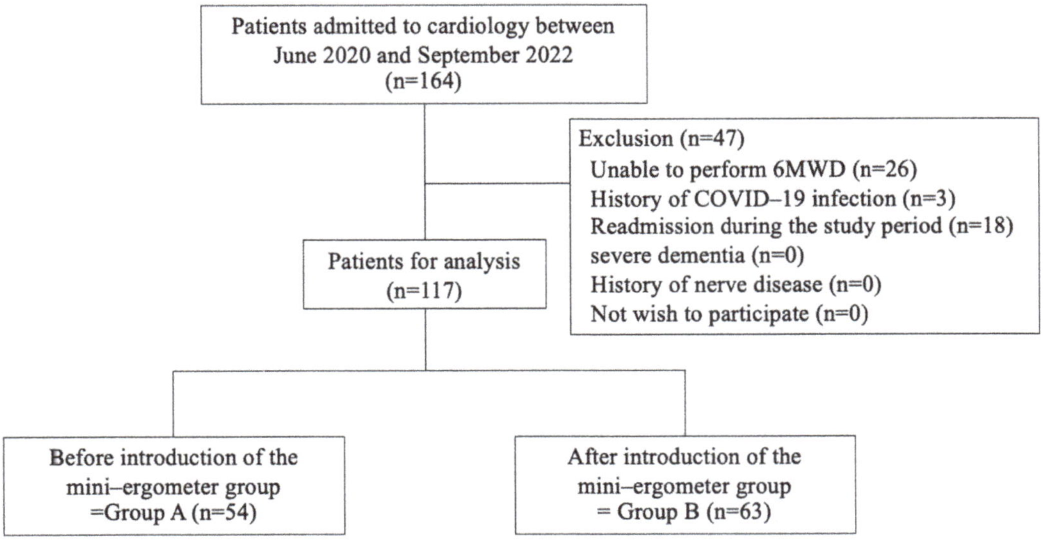

Figure 2. Patient flowchart.

Table 1. Patients' demographic and clinical characteristics at admission before and after the introduction of the mini-ergometer.

	Before the Introduction of the Mini-Ergometer (Group A) (n = 54)	After the Introduction of the Mini-Ergometer (Group B) (n = 63)	p
Age, years	83.0 (73.0–88.3)	84.0 (73.0–87.0)	0.540
Gender (male/female), n	28/26	34/29	0.819
Body mass index, kg/m^2	21.3 (18.1–23.6)	22.3 (19.7–24.7)	0.124
NYHA functional class			
Class I	7	8	0.966
Class II	26	22	0.147
Class III	16	27	0.139
Class IV	5	6	0.961
Comorbidities			
Hypertension	32	44	0.232
Dyslipidemia	14	22	0.293
Diabetes Mellitus	17	32	0.035
Myocardial Infarction	9	16	0.251
Cerebral Infarction	9	14	0.451
Cerebral Hemorrhage	2	3	0.778
Cancer	9	14	0.451
Chronic Kidney Disease	14	11	0.265
Medication			
Renin-angiotensin system inhibitor	12	3	0.863
Beta blocker	35	46	0.338
Calcium channel blocker	12	16	0.688
Loop diuretic	46	46	0.109
Thiazide diuretic	0	1	0.353
V2 receptor antagonist	21	32	0.197
Mineralocorticoid Receptor Antagonist	15	26	0.127
sodium-glucose cotransporter 2 inhibitor	8	15	0.222
Days before the initiation of the rehabilitation program, days	2.5 (2.0–4.3)	3.0 (2.0–4.0)	0.188
Length of hospitalization, days	19.0 (14.0–29.5)	18.0 (14.0–24.0)	0.749
Rehabilitation place, min	1310/185 (87.6/12.4)	1351/196 (87.3/12.5)	0.806
Ward	720.0 (420.0–1425.0)	660.0 (390.0–840.0)	0.109
Rehabilitation center	40.0 (0–120.0)	60.0 (0–180.0)	0.163
SBP, mmHg	139.0 (120.0–161.0)	136.0 (120.0–160.0)	0.716
NT-proBNP, pg/dL	5103 (2847–10,097)	3392 (1773–7034)	0.052
GNRI	94.5 (84.1–101.0)	95.5 (83.5–102.9)	0.707
Serum hemoglobin, g/dL	11.7 (10.2–13.5)	12.2 (10.6–13.6)	0.202
Serum albumin, g/dL	3.6 (3.2–3.9)	3.6 (3.3–3.9)	0.695
Serum sodium, mEq/L	141.0 (137.5–144.0)	140.0 (138.0–143.0)	0.541
eGFR, ml/min/1.73 m^2	47.2 (38.6–61.1)	50.0 (36.1–62.6)	0.688
LVEF, %	41.7 (29.9–60.1)	38.3 (27.9–55.8)	0.330
Grip strength, kg	18.3 (13.9–23.0)	19.3 (14.9–25.9)	0.367
Walking speed, m/s *	0.9 (0.7–1.0)	0.7 (0.5–0.9)	0.065
FIM score, points			
Total	97.5 (78.0–114.0)	105.0 (86.0–120.0)	0.153
Motor	69.0 (53.3–79.0)	71.0 (57.0–85.0)	0.141
Cognitive	35.0 (25.0–35.0)	35.0 (28.0–35.0)	0.190

FIM, Functional Independence Measure; GNRI, geriatric nutritional risk index; eGFR, estimated glomerular filtration rate; LVEF, left ventricular ejection fraction; NT-proBNP, N-terminal pro-brain natriuretic peptide; NYHA, New York Heart Association; SBP, systolic blood pressure. * The walking speed was calculated using the usual 10 m walk test.

Table 2 shows the patients' clinical characteristics at discharge. Group B showed a significantly higher 6MWD (Group A: 236.0 m vs. Group B: 290.0 m, $p = 0.020$) and a higher walking speed than Group A at discharge (Group A: 0.8 m/s vs. Group B: 0.9 m/s, $p = 0.084$).

Table 2. Patients' clinical characteristics at discharge before and after the introduction of the mini ergometer.

	Before the Introduction of the Mini-Ergometer (Group A) (*n* = 54)	After the Introduction of the Mini-Ergometer (Group B) (*n* = 63)	*p*
Grip strength, kg	18.5 (13.3–24.8)	21.0 (14.9–27.1)	0.163
Walking speed, m/s	0.8 (0.6–1.0)	0.9 (0.7–1.1)	0.084
Waist circumference, cm	81.0 (72.0–88.5)	85.1 (74.5–91.9)	0.178
KEMS, N/kg	3.3 (2.6–4.2)	3.6 (2.5–4.3)	0.779
6MWD, m	236.0 (163.8–312.5)	290.0 (214.5–350.0)	0.020
FRT, cm	26.0 (19.8–33.5)	30.0 (23.0–33.3)	0.144
MMSE-J	27.0 (22.0–28.5)	26.0 (23.0–28.0)	0.758
FIM score			
Total	114.5 (95.8–125.3)	120.0 (108.0–125.0)	0.154
Motor	80.5 (70.0–90.3)	85.0 (76.0–90.0)	0.153
Cognitive	35.0 (25.0–35.0)	35.0 (31.0–35.0)	0.105
FIM gain	11.5 (0–23.0)	8.0 (0–25.0)	0.949
FIM efficiency	0.5 (0–0.9)	0.5 (0–0.8)	0.920

Data were presented as median (interquartile range). FIM, Functional Independence Measure; FRT, functional reach test; KEMS, knee extensor muscle strength; MMSE, Mini-Mental State Examination; 6MWD, 6 min walking distance.

Regarding duration of the rehabilitation program during admission, Group B showed a significantly longer ergometer exercise time than Group A (Group A: 0 min vs. Group B: 25.0 min, $p < 0.001$). Group B showed a significantly shorter exercise time for range of motion, sitting, and standing exercises than Group A (range of motion exercise: Group A: 40.0 min vs. Group B: 0 min, $p < 0.001$; sitting exercise: Group A: 0 min vs. Group B: 0 min, $p = 0.019$; standing exercise: Group A: 5.0 min vs. Group B: 0 min, $p = 0.003$) (Table 3).

Table 3. Duration (min) of the rehabilitation program during admission. Data were presented as median (interquartile range). ADL, activities of daily living.

	Before the Introduction of the Mini-Ergometer (Group A) (*n* = 54)	After the Introduction of the Mini-Ergometer (Group B) (*n* = 63)	*p*
Assessment	250.0 (195.0–340.0)	260.0 (193.8–306.3)	0.600
Range of motion exercise	40.0 (8.8–107.5)	0 (0–25.0)	<0.001
Sitting up exercise	0 (0–0)	0 (0–0)	0.556
Sitting exercise	0 (0–35.0)	0 (0–0)	0.019
Standing exercise	5.0 (0–50.0)	0 (0–5.0)	0.003
Walking exercise	180.0 (81.3–402.5)	180.0 (100.0–280.0)	0.382
Ergometer exercise	0 (0–2.5)	25.0 (0–70.0)	<0.001
Resistance training	165.0 (78.8–327.5)	150.0 (95.0–240.0)	0.392
ADL training	0 (0–55.0)	0 (0–20.0)	0.313
Others	27.5 (5.0–67.5)	10.0 (0–30.0)	0.035
Total	790.0 (535.0–1550.0)	720.0 (480.0–940.0)	0.141

4. Discussion

With restricted access to rehabilitation centers during the COVID-19 pandemic, developing ways to maintain exercise quality and improve physical function during hospitalization was crucial. This study showed a statistically lower tendency in walking speed at the start of cardiac rehabilitation in patients with heart failure after the introduction of the mini-ergometer. However, a rather "higher" walking speed and a higher 6MWD at discharge were observed after the introduction of the mini-ergometer than before the introduction.

The results of this study showed a significantly higher 6MWD after the introduction of the mini-ergometer than before the introduction. The mini-ergometer has (1) the advantage of improving exercise tolerance [4,5], (2) improving walking speed [6], and (3) enhancing muscle strength [7]. The use of a mini-ergometer allowed for the quantification of exercise load, even when access to the rehabilitation center was limited. The introduction of the mini-ergometer might have contributed to the ability to perform sufficient aerobic exercise, which could contribute to the higher 6MWD at discharge. The ability to use a mini-ergometer in a confined space was a factor that allowed sufficient aerobic exercise at the appropriate intensity. In our hospital, aerobic exercise was mainly performed using ergometers before the COVID-19 outbreak. However, aerobic exercise could not be conducted under the restrictions on the rehabilitation center during the early phase of the pandemic. Therefore, the introduction of the mini-ergometer to the ward allowed sufficient time to be dedicated to aerobic exercise. This study showed a tendency toward a higher walking speed after the introduction of the mini-ergometer, which is consistent with previous studies, which reported improvements in walking speed after the use of the mini-ergometer [6]. Taken together, our method might improve physical function at discharge. No significant differences were observed between the groups in terms of age or MMSE-J scores. Previous studies focusing on patients with arterial hypertension have demonstrated that age exerts a significant negative impact on MMSE scores [20]. However, although the patients in both groups of the present study were of advanced age, their MMSE-J scores remained within the normal range.

The statement issued by the Japanese Society of Cardiac Rehabilitation defines it as follows: "Cardiac rehabilitation refers to a long-term, multifaceted, comprehensive program designed to optimize a cardiac patient's physical, psychological, social, and vocational status, in addition to stabilizing, slowing, or even reversing the progression of the underlying atherosclerotic or heart failure processes, thereby reducing recurrence, rehospitalization and mortality and enabling patients to live comfortably and actively. Cardiac rehabilitation programs include "medical assessment, prescribed exercise training, coronary risk factor modification, patient education, counseling and optimal medical therapy" for individual patients, which are provided by a multidisciplinary team in a coordinated manner [21]." Thus, although cardiac rehabilitation necessitates a multifaceted approach, pharmacological therapy is of particular importance in the acute-phase management of patients with heart failure [22]. It is therefore desirable to provide effective and efficient exercise therapy in conjunction with pharmacological interventions.

Because the provision of cardiac rehabilitation has been restricted due to the COVID-19 pandemic, efforts were needed to ensure that exercise therapy conducted in the ward maintained the same quality as that performed in the rehabilitation center [11,14]. In the rehabilitation program before the introduction of the mini-ergometer, a significant amount of time was spent on a range of motion, sitting, and standing exercises. Designing a rehabilitation program that can serve as an alternative to the ergometer within a confined space of a ward may be challenging. Aerobic exercise without the use of exercise equipment is typically represented by walking [8]. However, in this study, no significant difference in the treatment time of walking exercises for cardiac rehabilitation programs was observed between the two groups. Walking exercises conducted in the ward were sometimes performed as part of the mobilization assessment. Therefore, there might not be enough space in the ward for walking as an aerobic exercise. Since the mini-ergometer does not take up much space, a mini-ergometer was introduced to the ward to provide tailored quantitative and effective exercise prescriptions according to the patients' condition and physical function. Indeed, its utility in improving physical function in patients with heart failure has been demonstrated.

The social isolation due to the COVID-19 pandemic gradually eased, and life was slowly returning to normal. However, prolonged social isolation might negatively affect the current physical function in older patients with heart failure, as evidenced by the decreased walking speed observed in this study. Patients with heart failure who have a decline in physical function, including walking speed, have been reported to have a poor prognosis in terms of death and readmission [23,24]. The location for cardiac rehabilitation exercise was restricted due to the COVID-19 pandemic. Therefore, taking measures to ensure that the exercise content was not restricted was necessary.

During the COVID-19 pandemic, various lifestyle diseases were affected, such as the deterioration of diabetes control [25]. Additionally, cardiovascular diseases increased [26,27]. Therefore, the role of cardiac rehabilitation is significant. In this study, the rehabilitation methodology is considered highly important and valuable for future infectious disease outbreaks and disasters.

This study has some limitations. First, this was a single-center registry and retrospective study with a small sample size. Second, the different circumstances surrounding the healthcare systems in Japan and other countries might limit the generalizability of the study's results. Third, the baseline 6MWD was not measured. Therefore, the effect of the mini-ergometer could not be discussed. However, the findings highlighted the importance of implementing measures to maintain the quality of exercise intensity even when access to rehabilitation centers is limited during pandemics.

5. Conclusions

The findings of this study demonstrate that the introduction of a mini-ergometer to the ward could ensure quantitative exercise intensity even under restrictions on access to rehabilitation centers during the COVID-19 outbreak, leading to improvements in physical function (6MWD, Walking speed) at discharge in patients with heart failure. The rehabilitation methodology is regarded as highly important and valuable for addressing future infectious disease outbreaks and disasters.

Author Contributions: Conceptualization, E.M. and H.I.; methodology, E.M., H.I. and H.K.; software, E.W. and H.M.; validation, E.M., R.S., T.H., Y.S. and E.W.; formal analysis, E.M. and Y.K.; investigation, R.S. and T.H.; resources, Y.A. and H.K.; data curation, E.M.; writing—original draft preparation, E.M., H.I. and H.M.; writing—review and editing, Y.K., Y.A., R.S., T.H.,Y.S., E.W. and H.K.; visualization, E.M.; supervision, H.I. and H.K.; project administration, H.K. All authors have read and agreed to the published version of the manuscript.

Funding: This work was supported in part by JSPS KAKENHI Grant Number 24K20546.

Institutional Review Board Statement: The study was conducted in accordance with the Declaration of Helsinki, and approved by the Research Ethics Committee of Fujita Health University(Approval No.: HM20-538, 30 March 2021).

Informed Consent Statement: Informed consent was obtained from all subjects using the opt-out method, which was approved by the Committee.

Data Availability Statement: The data that support the findings of this study are available from the corresponding author upon reasonable request.

Conflicts of Interest: Eiichi Watanabe is a consultant to Fukuda Denshi. The other authors declare no conflicts of interest.

Abbreviations

The following abbreviations are used in this manuscript:

6MWD	6 min walking distance
ADL	activities of daily living
KEMS	knee extensor muscle strength
FIM	Functional Independence Measure
GNRI	geriatric nutritional risk index
eGFR	estimated glomerular filtration rate
LVEF	left ventricular ejection fraction
NT-pro BNP	N-terminal pro-brain natriuretic peptide
NYHA	New York Heart Association
SBP	systolic blood pressure
FRT	functional reach test
MMSE	Mini-Mental State Examination

References

1. Fletcher, G.F.; Balady, G.; Blair, S.N.; Blumenthal, J.; Caspersen, C.; Chaitman, B.; Epstein, S.; Froelicher, E.S.S.; Froelicher, V.F.; Pina, I.L.; et al. Statement on exercise: Benefits and recommendations for physical activity programs for all Americans. A statement for health professionals by the Committee on Exercise and Cardiac Rehabilitation of the Council on Clinical Cardiology, American Heart Association. *Circulation* **1996**, *94*, 857–862. [CrossRef] [PubMed]
2. Haykowsky, M.J.; Liang, Y.; Pechter, D.; Jones, L.W.; McAlister, F.A.; Clark, A.M. A meta-analysis of the effect of exercise training on left ventricular remodeling in heart failure patients: The benefit depends on the type of training performed. *J. Am. Coll. Cardiol.* **2007**, *49*, 2329–2336. [CrossRef]
3. Belardinelli, R.; Georgiou, D.; Cianci, G.; Purcaro, A. Randomized, controlled trial of long-term moderate exercise training in chronic heart failure: Effects on functional capacity, quality of life, and clinical outcome. *Circulation* **1999**, *9*, 1173–1182. [CrossRef] [PubMed]
4. Noguchi, M.; Miyagi, S.; Moroe, M.; Yamaguchi, S.; Koshino, Y. Effects of intradialytic exercise intervention with paced constant pedal rates in hemodialysis patients. *Rigakuryoho Kagaku* **2017**, *32*, 73–80. (In Japanese) [CrossRef]
5. Burtin, C.; Clerckx, B.; Robbeets, C.; Ferdinande, P.; Langer, D.; Troosters, T.; Hermans, G.; Decramer, M.; Gosselink, R. Early exercise in critically ill patients enhances short-term functional recovery. *Crit. Care Med.* **2009**, *37*, 2499–2505. [CrossRef]
6. Veldema, J.; Bösl, K.; Kugler, P.; Ponfick, M.; Gdynia, H.J.; Nowak, D.A. Cycle ergometer training vs. resistance training in ICU-acquired weakness. *Acta Neurol. Scand.* **2019**, *140*, 62–71. [CrossRef] [PubMed]
7. Harris, S.; LeMaitre, J.P.; Mackenzie, G.; Fox, K.A.; Denvir, M.A. A randomised study of home-based electrical stimulation of the legs and conventional bicycle exercise training for patients with chronic heart failure. *Eur. Heart J.* **2003**, *24*, 871–878. [CrossRef]
8. Makita, S.; Yasu, T.; Akashi, Y.J.; Adachi, H.; Izawa, H.; Ishihara, S.; Iso, Y.; Ohuchi, H.; Omiya, K.; Ohya, Y.; et al. JCS/JACR 2021 guideline on rehabilitation in patients with cardiovascular disease. *Circ. J.* **2022**, *87*, 155–235. [CrossRef]
9. Ozemek, C.; Berry, R.; Bonikowske, A.R.; German, C.; Gavic, A.M. What has cardiac rehabilitation looked like in the COVID-19 pandemic: Lessons learned for the future. *Prog. Cardiovasc. Dis.* **2023**, *76*, 20–24. [CrossRef]
10. Ghisi, G.L.M.; Xu, Z.; Liu, X.; Mola, A.; Gallagher, R.; Babu, A.S.; Yeung, C.; Marzolini, S.; Buckley, J.; Oh, P.; et al. Impacts of the COVID-19 Pandemic on Cardiac Rehabilitation Delivery around the World. *Glob. Heart* **2021**, *16*, 43. [CrossRef]
11. Kida, K.; Nishitani-Yokoyama, M.; Oishi, S.; Kono, Y.; Kamiya, K.; Kishi, T.; Node, K.; Makita, S.; Kimura, Y. Japanese Association of Cardiac Rehabilitation (JACR) Public Relations Committee. Nationwide Survey of Japanese cardiac rehabilitation training facilities during the coronavirus disease 2019 outbreak. *Circ. Rep.* **2021**, *3*, 311–315. [CrossRef]
12. Izawa, H.; Yoshida, T.; Ikegame, T.; Izawa, K.P.; Ito, Y.; Okamura, H.; Osada, N.; Kinugawa, S.; Kubozono, T.; Kono, Y.; et al. Japanese association of cardiac rehabilitation standard cardiac rehabilitation program planning committee. Standard cardiac rehabilitation program for heart failure. *Circ. J.* **2019**, *83*, 2394–2398. [CrossRef]
13. World Health Organization. Avoid the Three CS. Available online: https://www.who.int/brunei/news/infographics{-}{-}-english (accessed on 5 March 2021).
14. Aoyagi, Y.; Mori, E.; Ishii, H.; Kono, Y.; Sato, A.; Okochi, Y.; Funahashi, R.; Kagaya, H. Poor walking ability outcome and activities of daily living improvement in patients undergoing cardiac rehabilitation during COVID-19 pandemic. *Eur. J. Phys. Rehabil. Med.* **2022**, *58*, 606–611. [CrossRef]

15. Yamada, K.; Furuya, R.; Takita, T.; Maruyama, Y.; Yamaguchi, Y.; Ohkawa, S.; Kumagai, H. Simplified nutritional screening tools for patients on maintenance hemodialysis. *Am. J. Clin. Nutr.* **2008**, *87*, 106–113. [CrossRef] [PubMed]
16. ATS Committee on Proficiency Standards for Clinical Pulmonary Function Laboratories. ATS statement: Guidelines for the six-minute walk test. *Am. J. Respir. Crit. Care Med.* **2002**, *166*, 111–117. [CrossRef] [PubMed]
17. Morio, Y.; Omori, Y.; Izawa, K.; Tanaka, A.; Watanabe, S.; Beppu, M.; Kawama, K. The development of Functional Reach Test using the telescoping rod. *Sogo Rehabil.* **2007**, *35*, 487–493. (In Japanese)
18. Sugishita, M.; Hemmi, I. Validity and reliability of mini mental state examination-japanese (MMSE–J): A preliminary report. *Jpn. J. Cogn Neurosci.* **2010**, *12*, 186–190. (In Japanese) [CrossRef]
19. Granger, C.V.; Hamilton, B.B.; Linacre, J.M.; Heinemann, A.W.; Wright, B.D. Performance profiles of the functional independence measure. *Am. J. Phys. Med. Rehabil.* **1993**, *72*, 84–89. [CrossRef]
20. Kapusta, J.; Kidawa, T.M.; Rynkowska-Kidawa, M.; IrzmaŃski, T.R.; Kowalski, T.J. Evaluation of frequency of occurrence of cognitive impairment in the course of arterial hypertension in an elderly population. *Psychogeriatrics* **2020**, *20*, 406–411. [CrossRef]
21. JACR Statement. Mission of the Japanese Association of Cardiac Rehabilitation. 2013. Available online: https://www.jacr.jp/cms/wp-content/uploads/2015/04/statement.pdf (accessed on 25 January 2013).
22. Mauriello, A.; Ascrizzi, A.; Roma, A.S.; Molinari, R.; Caturano, A.; Imbalzano, E.; D'Andrea, A.; Russo, V. Effects of Heart Failure Therapies on Atrial Fibrillation: Biological and Clinical Perspectives. *Antioxidants* **2024**, *13*, 806. [CrossRef]
23. Pulignano, G.; Del Sindaco, D.; Di Lenarda, A.; Alunni, G.; Senni, M.; Tarantini, L.; Cioffi, G.; Tinti, M.D.; Barbati, G.; Minardi, G.; et al. IMAGE-HF Study Investigators. Incremental value of gait speed in predicting prognosis of older adults with heart failure: Insights from the IMAGE-HF study. *JACC Heart Fail.* **2016**, *4*, 289–298. [CrossRef]
24. Tanaka, S.; Kamiya, K.; Hamazaki, N.; Matsuzawa, R.; Nozaki, K.; Nakamura, T.; Yamashita, M.; Maekawa, E.; Noda, C.; Yamaoka-Tojo, M.; et al. Short-term change in gait speed and clinical outcomes in older patients with acute heart failure. *Circ. J.* **2019**, *83*, 1860–1867. [CrossRef] [PubMed]
25. Tanji, Y.; Sawada, S.; Watanabe, T.; Mita, T.; Kobayashi, Y.; Murakami, T.; Metoki, H.; Akai, H. Impact of COVID-19 pandemic on glycemic control among outpatients with type 2 diabetes in Japan: A hospital-based survey from a country without lockdown. *Diabetes Res. Clin. Pract.* **2021**, *176*, 108840. [CrossRef]
26. Ministry of Health, Labour and Welfare. Provides an Overview of Key Vital Statistics in Japan for 2022. Available online: https://www.mhlw.go.jp/toukei/saikin/hw/jinkou/geppo/nengai22/dl/gaikyouR4.pdf (accessed on 1 June 2023).
27. Tanaka, H.; Togawa, K.; Katanoda, K. Impact of the COVID-19 pandemic on mortality trends in Japan: A reversal in 2021? A descriptive analysis of national mortality data, 1995–2021. *BMJ Open* **2023**, *13*, e071785. [CrossRef]

Journal of
Clinical Medicine

MDPI

Review

How to Evaluate and Adjust the Recommended Level of Physical Activity in Patients with Congenital Heart Diseases? A Practical Approach

Dominika Filipiak-Strzecka [1], Ibadete Bytyçi [2,3] and Agata Bielecka-Dabrowa [1,4,*]

1 Department of Cardiology and Congenital Heart Diseases of Adults, Polish Mother's Memorial Hospital Research Institute (PMMHRI), 93-338 Lodz, Poland; dominika.filipiak-strzecka@iczmp.edu.pl
2 Medical Faculty, University of Prishtina, 10000 Prishtina, Kosovo
3 Clinic of Cardiology, University Clinical Centre of Kosovo, 10000 Prishtina, Kosovo
4 Department of Preventive Cardiology and Lipidology, Medical University of Lodz, 93-338 Lodz, Poland
* Correspondence: agata.bielecka-dabrowa@iczmp.edu.pl; Tel.: +48-422-711-591

Abstract: The prolongation of the lifespan of patients with congenital heart diseases (CHD) has caused them to experience symptoms and complications not only related to the defect itself or late complications of surgical treatment but also to be at risk of population diseases such as obesity or ischemic heart disease. As recently as two decades ago, fewer than one in five CHD patients received formal advice on physical activity. Once a patient has been thoroughly evaluated and the risk has been stratified, the clinician can develop a detailed and individualized exercise prescription. This prescription is a formal plan that specifies the recommended frequency, intensity, duration, and type of physical activity. The goal is to maximize the health benefits of exercise while minimizing any potential risks. Although the anatomical classification of the defect and the previously implemented method of treatment allow the estimation of the possible late complications to a certain extent, in reality, the clinician condition may vary significantly in individual cases. For this reason, we prepared a practical approach regarding physical activity in patients with CHD based on hemodynamic and electrophysiological parameters, instead of focusing solely on specific defects. We also paid attention to special CHD patient populations in which separate indications regarding physical activity must be implemented.

Keywords: congenital heart diseases; physical activity; exercise testing

1. Introduction

With the constant development of medicine and the much-needed improvement of care for children with congenital heart diseases (CHDs) in recent decades, survival to adulthood in this group has significantly increased [1–5]. Thus, in developed countries, treatment of patients with CHD is no longer the exclusive domain of pediatric cardiologists but also involves adult cardiology specialists [6]. Currently, this population consists mostly of adult patients [3]. The prolongation of the lifespan of patients with CHD has caused them to experience symptoms and complications not only related to the defect itself or late complications of surgical treatment but also to be at risk of population diseases such as obesity or ischemic heart disease [7,8]. The prevalence of CAD in ACHD patients is higher than in the general population [9]. Arterial hypertension is also more often diagnosed in CHD group, with the prevalence varying between 30 and 50% [8,10]. Obesity and overweight are at least as common amongst patients with congenital heart disease as in the general population [11,12]. On the brighter side, possibly due to health education, the proportion of ACHD patients who smoke has been reported to be smaller than in the general population [9,11].

It is well established that in the general population, to reduce the risk of developing these diseases, regular physical activity is recommended. This might be in stark contrast with traditional circumstances, due to which patients with CHD encounter parental and environmental overprotection, often resulting in reduced physical activity. As recently as two decades ago, fewer than one in five CHD patients received formal advice on physical activity [13]. Meanwhile, there has been emerging evidence regarding the benefits of physical exercise on cardiorespiratory fitness (CRF), prognosis, quality of life, and psychosocial health in patients with CHD [14]. The ESC and AHA guidelines strongly support the claim that the topic of physical activity should be discussed during each visit [5]. On the other hand, a vastly different anatomy and physiology of the heart of a CHD patient requires special attention and modification of existing recommendations created with the general population in mind [15]. Although the anatomical classification of the defect and the previously implemented method of treatment allow the estimation of possible late complications to a certain extent, in reality, the clinical condition may vary significantly in individual cases. For this reason, the current recommendations regarding physical activity in patients with CHD are based on hemodynamic and electrophysiological parameters, instead of focusing solely on specific defects [15].

2. Material and Methods

The aim of our study was to create a practical guide aiding clinicians in counseling adult congenital heart defect patients in terms of possible and desired levels of physical activity as this area of cardiologic care appears to be relatively uncovered.

An electronic search was completed in MEDLINE, SCOPUS, and Cochrane Database of Systematic Reviews according to existing guidelines pertaining to the topic. Recommendations were extracted and assembled from the identified articles to formulate a set of suggestions.

Databases were searched by using the following keywords: congenital heart diseases; congenital heart defect; exercise prescription; training program; physical activity.

Results were limited to the articles published within the 2010–2025 timeframe to capture up-to-date information regarding the subject.

3. Before Recommendations Can Be Made—Patients' Condition Assessment

3.1. At Rest—Basic Methods

3.1.1. Echocardiography

Echocardiography is generally considered the first-line modality for cardiovascular imaging in adults with CHD. Oftentimes, it is a sufficient diagnostic tool not only for reliable evaluation of cardiac morphology but also function and hemodynamic relevance of the malformations.

Echocardiographic assessment should follow the published general guidelines [16,17] but needs to take into account the specifics of ventricular pathophysiology in certain CHDs such as the central role of the right ventricle (RV) or the presence of intracardiac or extracardiac shunts [18]. The most important parameters that require assessment are:

- Ventricle systolic function: left ventricle ejection fraction (LVEF), tricuspid annular plane systolic excursion (TAPSE), and fractional area change (FAC) for RV function, 3D echocardiography when feasible;
- LV/RV pressure load: left/right ventricular outflow tract (LVOT/RVOT) peak systolic velocity to assess the LVOT/RVOT gradient;

- LV/RV volume load: the presence of valve regurgitation or shunt, the presence of RV or LV dilatation (LV end diastolic volume—LV EDV, RV end diastolic area—RV EDA)
- Pulmonary pressure estimation; in most risk stratification scale tricuspid valve regurgitation velocity (TRV) was used; however, in certain clinical scenarios (e.g., excentric jet) where reliable TRV measurement is not possible, other parameters, such as acceleration time of the pulmonary valve or mid-systolic notching, early diastolic pulmonary regurgitation velocity, or pulmonary artery dilatation, should be taken into consideration. In particularly complicated cases, right heart catheterization should be considered a golden standard.
- Aortic diameters: the aortic root diameter, measured in the parasternal long axis view (as the short axis may underestimate the diameter due to possible plane obliquity); the ascending aorta diameter, measured in end-diastole in the parasternal long axis view, often 1–2 intercostal spaces up [15,19,20].

3.1.2. Arrythmia Detection: Resting ECG and 24-h (or Prolonged) ECG Monitoring

In CHD, arrhythmogenic substrates often arise from surgical scars, chamber dilation, pressure or volume overload, and long-standing myocardial remodeling rather than from acquired coronary or degenerative conduction system disease [21]. Atrial arrhythmias, such as intra-atrial reentrant tachycardia or atypical atrial flutter, are particularly prevalent in patients after atrial switch procedures or complex repairs involving extensive atriotomy. Ventricular arrhythmias may develop due to patch borders, fibrotic tissue, or residual outflow tract obstruction, as seen in repaired tetralogy of Fallot [22]. Moreover, conduction disturbances, including sinus node dysfunction and atrioventricular block, are common sequelae of surgical interventions or chronic hemodynamic stress. Unlike in the general population, where age-related fibrosis and ischemic injury predominate, arrhythmias in CHD often emerge at a younger age and may coexist with cyanosis, ventricular dysfunction, or pulmonary hypertension, significantly impacting exercise tolerance and prognosis [5]. A resting ECG can unveil conduction abnormalities, chamber enlargement, repolarization disturbances or accessory pathways, each of which may represent an arrhythmogenic substrate that could be unmasked or exacerbated by exertion [19,20]. Extended monitoring further allows detection of both symptomatic and silent supraventricular or ventricular arrhythmias. The assessment should be mostly focused on the prevalence of premature ventricular complex (PVC), coupled PVC, atrial fibrillation/atrial flutter, either non-sustained or sustained ventricular tachycardia [23]. Less than 500 PVC/24 h is considered clinically irrelevant [15]. In the case of arrythmia recognition, it is crucial to assess whether it worsens with exertion. When this initial testing fails to detect any significant abnormalities and there is a clinical suspicion of the arrythmia, further investigations, such as electrophysiology study or provocative tests, may be required. If the treatment is established and the clinical improvement is observed, re-assessment should be made to adjust the exercise prescription to the patient's current condition.

3.1.3. Assessment of Oxygen Saturation

Central cyanosis is largely excluded when transcutaneous saturations are higher than 95% at rest and during exercise. In patients with a potential right-to-left shunt, transcutaneous arterial saturation at rest should be recorded. Low arterial saturation due to pulmonary disease must not be overlooked [15].

3.2. *Exercise Testing—Cardiopulmonary Exercise Test (CPET)*

CPET enables objective measurement of the exercise capacity, which might be overestimated when self-reported by patients, may unmask impairments and arrhythmias even in asymptomatic patients, and is an integral part of the decision-making process [24]. CPET accompanied by 12-lead ECG is an important tool for assessing the baseline fitness of individuals and helps to choose the proper types of sport and level of intensity [25].

Most clinically valuable parameters to be assessed:

Cardiopulmonary indices:

Peak-oxygen consumption (peak VO_2)—most studied CPET variable in CHD [24] and is one of the best predictors of morbidity and mortality in patients with CHD [26,27]. The prognostic cut-off value in patients with CHD is considered ≤36% of predicted peak VO_2 [27]. However, serial decline may be more predictive than a single abnormal value [28]. Moreover, it is considered the most widely used measure of CRF. The spectrum of expected peak VO_2 values differs depending on the ailment [27–29].

Heart rate reserve (HRR)—prognostically significant in CHD patients, particularly in the presence of cyanosis. Low HRR is an independent predictor of adverse outcomes. Chronotropic incompetence is very common in CHD patients. HRR is a strong predictor of mortality, transplant risk, and hospitalization in patients with Fontann circulation [25].

Ventilatory efficiency VE/VCO_2 slope—useful parameter in the context of sub-maximal testing; often increased above the norm in patients with reduced LVEF, ventilation/perfusion mismatch, or right-to-left shunting. The prognostic cut-off value, predicting poor outcome in patients with CHD is >39 [27].

Ventilatory anaerobic threshold (VAT)—the most widely used measure of fitness during submaximal effort test, often decreased in CHD or deconditioning; according to the current guidelines distinction between the first and second ventilatory threshold (VT1 and VT2), it is recommended. VAT represents the same exertion stage as VT1 and marks the transition from purely aerobic to mixed aerobic–anaerobic metabolism. It also reflects the onset of lactate accumulation and bicarbonate buffering, which leads to a mild compensatory increase in ventilation [30,31].

Second ventilatory threshold (VT2, also termed as the anaerobic threshold) marks the intensity at which ventilation increases disproportionately relative to both VO_2 and VCO_2. This occurs when lactic acid production exceeds the buffering capacity of bicarbonate, causing metabolic acidosis. VT_2 represents the upper limit of sustainable exercise intensity, above which steady-state metabolism is no longer possible, and fatigue ensues rapidly [30,31].

O_2 pulse—decreased when impaired stroke volume or abnormalities in oxygen extraction is observed.

Arrhythmias—detection of arrhythmias during exercise increases the risk of sudden death by 6.6-fold [32].

Heart rate—measured continuously during exercise may reveal chronotropic incompetence, which in CHD patients, is often a symptom of ventricular dysfunction or ischemia [33].

Blood pressure—A normal blood pressure response during exercise includes a rise in systolic blood pressure by ≥25 mmHg, to a maximum of 220 mmHg (men) and 200 mmHg (women). An impaired response or a drop of systolic blood pressure during exercise should raise concern and be further diagnosed. The most common CPET abnormalities characteristic of different CHD phenotypes are summarized in Table 1.

Table 1. Main CPET parameters abnormalities in different CHD phenotypes. Adapted and simplified from Guglielmi G et al., 2025 [25].

CHD Type	Peak VO_2	VE/VCO_2 Slope	VAT	HRR
Biventricular circulation with systemic LV	~71% predicted;	Normal/mildly elevated	Often reduced	Frequently reduced.
Biventricular circulation with systemic RV	~63–67% predicted	Mildly elevated	Reduced	Frequently reduced;
Fontan circulation	~59% predicted	Mildly elevated	Reduced	Frequently reduced
Eisenmenger syndrome	~42% predicted	Significantly elevated	Markedly reduced	Frequently reduced

VAT—ventilatory anaerobic threshold; CHD—congenital heart disease; HRR—heart rate reserve production; LV—left ventricle; RV—right ventricle; VE/VCO_2—ventilation to carbon dioxide output; VO_2—oxygen uptake.

3.3. *Additional Assessment Methods—To Be Used in Specific Circumstances*

3.3.1. Cardiovascular Magnetic Resonance

Cardiovascular magnetic resonance (CMR) may be required to assess right and left ventricular (LV) volumes and function, myocardial scars (which may act as a surrogate for arrhythmia risk), regurgitant fraction, visualization of prosthetic materials (conduits), and detailed morphological studies (e.g., pulmonary veins, coronary arteries), which can all impact on ventricular function in patients with CHD [19].

Borderline or pathological aortic diameter values found in echocardiography require additional cross-sectional imaging by CT or CMR.

3.3.2. Computed Tomography

Computed tomography (CT) is the imaging modality of choice for the delineation of small anatomical structures such as coronary arteries and collateral arteries and for imaging parenchymal lung pathology [19].

Borderline or pathological aortic diameter values found in echocardiography require additional cross-sectional imaging by CT or CMR.

3.3.3. Right Heart Catheterization

RHC provides precise measurements of intracardiac pressures, cardiac output, pulmonary and systemic vascular resistance, and oxygen saturations [5]. In CHD patients, RHC is particularly valuable for evaluating the severity and reversibility of pulmonary hypertension, quantifying intracardiac shunts, and assessing the hemodynamic impact of residual or complex lesions such as conduit stenosis, intracardiac shunts, or single-ventricle physiology [34]. In everyday clinical practice, RHC is usually recommended when the results of noninvasive diagnostic methods are inconclusive or not sufficient, such as in patients with a high echocardiographic probability of pulmonary hypertension, especially when considering limiting the practice of some or all sports, including competitive sports [19]. One has to keep in mind that RHC in CHD patients requires tailored protocols and experienced operators due to the heterogeneous anatomy, previous surgical repairs, and frequent presence of collateral vessels or baffles [35].

3.3.4. Spirometry

Evaluation with spirometry should be included in patients with reduced arterial saturation without a cardiovascular explanation [15,19].

3.3.5. Implantable Loop Recorder and an Electrophysiology Study

In patients with a high risk of arrythmia, especially in competitive athletes, additional methods of arrythmia assessment may be required before the final decision regarding physical activity is made [19].

3.3.6. Coronary Artery Disease Diagnostic Methods–Imaging, Exercise Test and Coronarography

In the case of coronary artery disease suspicion, the diagnostic path for the general population is usually recommended. It is worth mentioning that even significant coronary artery disease can be symptomless in patients with a congenital heart defect, who underwent surgical treatment due to a possible partial denervation as a consequence of the procedure [36]. For this reason, a routine exercise test should be considered before an exercise prescription can be made. In the case of the signs of inducible myocardial ischemia, the invasive coronarography might be necessary to assess the risk and indication for revascularization [20]. The special high-risk group of premature coronary artery disease includes patients with coarctation of the aorta (CoA) and patients after coronary replacement, e.g., surgically treated transposition of the great arteries [36]. From a clinical viewpoint, it is essential to postpone physical activity recommendations until non-invasive coronary artery disease diagnostics are performed. In the case of an anomalous origin of coronary artery disease, imaging (invasive or noninvasive angiography) is used to rule out the malignant anatomical type of the anomaly, and exercise testing is recommended. In the case of high-risk anatomical conditions (e.g., acute angled take-off from the aorta resulting in a slit-like orifice with reduced lumen and anomalous coursing between the aorta and the pulmonary artery) or exercise-induced ischemia, only low-intensity skill sports may be allowed prior to surgical correction [20].

4. Physical Activity Prescription

The process of risk profiling involves integrating the findings from the medical history, physical examination, cardiac imaging, and, most importantly, the objective exercise test. This synthesis allows the clinician to classify the patient into a general risk category—typically low, moderate, or high. A critical function of the risk stratification process is to identify absolute and relative contraindications to certain types of physical activity. The presence of specific "red flag" conditions necessitates significant activity restriction and, in some cases, may preclude participation in all but the lowest intensity activities [37]. The specific parameters determining the risk category classification are presented in Figure 1.

Once a patient has been thoroughly evaluated and the risk has been stratified, the clinician can develop a detailed and individualized exercise prescription. This prescription is a formal plan that specifies the recommended frequency, intensity, duration, and type of physical activity. The goal is to maximize the health benefits of exercise while minimizing any potential risks. The FITT-VP principle (Frequency, Intensity, Time, Type, Volume, and Progression) provides a comprehensive framework for structuring this prescription [38]. The main recommendations, taking into account the established level of risk in the CHD patients, in accordance with FITT-VP principles, are presented in Table 2.

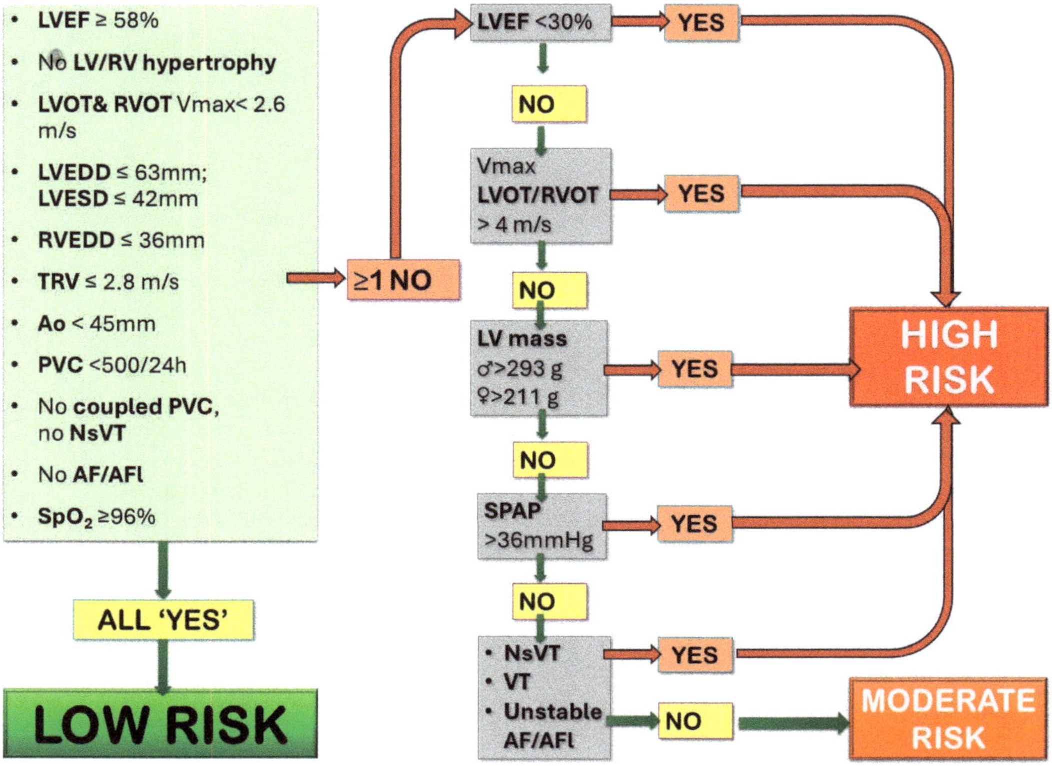

Figure 1. A flowchart helping to determine the recommended exercise level for patients with congenital heart disease. On the basis of Budts et al., Eur Heart J 2013 [15]. AF—atrial fibrillation; AFL—atrial fluttering; Ao—aorta; LV—left ventricle; LVEDD—left ventricular end diastolic diameter; LVESD—left ventricular end systolic diameter; LVEF—left ventricular ejection fraction; LVOT—left ventricular outflow tract; NsVT—non-sustained ventricular tachycardia; PVC-RV—right ventricle; RVEDD—right ventricular end diastolic diameter; RVOT—right ventricular outflow tract; SpO_2—oxygen saturation; SPAP—systolic pulmonary artery pressure; TVRV—tricuspid regurgitation velocity; VT—ventricular tachycardia.

Table 2. FITT-VP principle application for different CHD risk categories [20,38–40]. RPE—rate of perceived exertion; VAT—ventilatory anaerobic threshold; VT1—first ventilatory threshold.

FITT-VP Component	Low Risk	Moderate Risk	High Risk (Medically Supervised)
Frequency	5–7 days/week	3–5 days/week	3–5 days/week
Intensity (Aerobic)	Moderate to vigorous. RPE 13–17. Can progress to activity above VAT/VT1 or even VT2.	Low to Moderate. RPE 11–14. Generally maintain activity between VAT/VT1 and VT2.	Low. RPE 9–11. Activity must remain below VAT/VT1. Continuous monitoring may be required.
Time (Duration)	30–60 min per session.	20–40 min per session. May start with 10–15 min bouts.	15–30 min per session. Start with short bouts (5–10 min) with frequent rest periods.
Type	Wide variety of aerobic and recreational sports. Competitive sports often permissible after evaluation.	Rhythmic, large muscle group activities (e.g., walking, cycling, swimming). Avoid high-intensity competitive sports.	Low-impact, low-intensity activities (e.g., slow walking, light cycling, water aerobics).

Table 2. *Cont.*

FITT-VP Component	Low Risk	Moderate Risk	High Risk (Medically Supervised)
Volume	Aim for ≥150 min moderate or ≥75 min vigorous activity/week.	Gradually work toward 150 min moderate activity/week.	Volume is secondary to safety; focus on consistency and gradual progression of duration at low intensity.
Progression	Gradual increase in intensity and duration as tolerated.	Slow and gradual progression. Increase duration before intensity. Re-evaluate before progressing to vigorous activity.	Very slow progression under medical guidance. Any change requires re-evaluation.
Resistance Training	2–3 days/week. Moderate intensity.	2 days/week. Low intensity, higher repetitions (12–15). Avoid Valsalva maneuver.	1 to 2 days/week. Very low intensity, focusing on activities of daily living. May require supervision.

4.1. Types of Physical Effort Activities

4.1.1. Aerobic Training

Most studies concerning patients with congenital heart disease have focused on aerobic (endurance) exercises training (ET). Aerobic training (e.g., walking, cycling, swimming) primarily increases the cardiac output via augmented stroke volume and heart rate, improving peak VO_2, endothelial function, insulin sensitivity, and overall quality of life [20].

The minimum threshold of aerobic exercise intensity for patients with congenital heart disease (CHD) remains insufficiently defined, and absolute intensity prescriptions differ considerably depending on the underlying defect and the individual's baseline CRF. Exercise programs frequently determine aerobic training intensity from maximal heart rate (HRmax) obtained during exercise testing. Most interventions apply workloads within 60–80% of HRmax [41–43]; however, studies have also reported effective protocols at intensities as low as 40% of HRmax [44] and as high as 95% of HRmax, the latter typically within interval training regimens.

Recent findings indicate that high-intensity interval training (HIIT) may safely enhance CRF in adults with congenital heart disease (CHD). A systematic review encompassing 3 studies and 87 adults found no serious adverse events and noted improvements in peak oxygen uptake among participants undergoing HIIT regimens [45]. Additional data from a randomized controlled trial in adults with the corrected tetralogy of Fallot demonstrated that interval training significantly improved VO_2-peak, vascular endothelial function, and biomarkers like NT-proBNP and fibrinogen [46]. Although randomized studies remain limited, this emerging evidence supports HIIT as a promising, lesion-specific intervention in CHD rehabilitation.

4.1.2. Resistance Training

Resistance training (e.g., machine or free-weight exercises, use of bands) produces a brief, higher afterload with less sustained tachycardia, which increases muscular strength, bone density, and functional capacity; when performed at light to moderate loads with avoidance of prolonged Valsalva, it has favorable hemodynamic profiles for many CHD patients.

The systematic review by Hao et al. showed a moderate improvement in muscle strength achieved with strength training alone, with a minor improvement in peak VO_2 in a group of patients with congenital heart disease. The most effective method for VO_2-peak improvement was combined strength training with inspiratory muscle training [47].

Rest intervals of approximately 60 s between sets are advised to permit normalization of blood pressure and heart rate. Resistance training should be initiated at low intensities and gradually progressed to reach target levels, with movements performed at a controlled tempo of 2/0/2 s (eccentric/isometric/concentric) [42]. To elicit clinically relevant muscle hypertrophy, a frequency of 2–3 non-consecutive sessions per week is generally required [48]. Exercise prescriptions should emphasize large functional muscle groups of both the upper and lower extremities, with particular attention to the lower limbs in individuals with Fontan physiology, where enhanced skeletal muscle pump activity may provide additional circulatory support [49,50].

4.2. How to Assess the Recommended Exercise Intensity?

Contemporary literature favors an individual approach and recommendations based on relative exercise intensity. For this purpose, the measured objective CPET values with particular emphasis on the maximal heart rate is essential. It was also confirmed that objective CPET parameters corelate well with subjective estimates such as the rate of perceived exertion (RPE).

Up-to-date position statement suggests determining the exercise intensity by assessing VT1 and VT2. Typically, 'ET zones' could then be established as low-intense (at an HR or workload below VT1)—a level which should not be exceeded in high-risk patient groups; moderate–intense (at an HR of workload between VT1 and VT2)—appropriate for moderate-risk groups; and high-intense (at an HR or workload above VT2)—which may be considered in low-risk groups. If VT cannot be traced due to technical constraints, clinicians may recommend the exercise intensity on the basis of the maximal heart rate (HRmax) achieved during CPET (low intense: <55% of HRmax, moderate intense: 55–74% of HRmax; high intense: 75% of HRmax or more) [30,31].

The RPE Borg scale is based on the patient's subjective sensations during a workout. Recommendations divide exercise load into three categories: low intensity (RPE Borg Scale 11–12)—light to moderate subjective description of exercise intensity with individual feelings of not exceeding light perspiring; moderate intensity—(RPE Borg Scale 13–14)—moderate to hard subjective description of exercise intensity with individual feelings of intensive perspiring to light sweating; high intensity—(RPE Borg Scale 15–17)—hard to very hard subjective description of exercise intensity with individual feelings of sweating and hard working [15].

Subjective assessment with the use of the Borg scale may be especially useful in CHD patients, in whom chronotropic incompetence or atrial fibrillation may be present and affecting the practical usefulness of a fixed percentage MHR application. In this group of patients, the basic estimation methods, like 'if you can talk while exercising' rule to approximate moderate relative exercise intensity, may prove helpful in everyday practice [51].

Recent advances in digital health have introduced new opportunities for remote and home-based management, which might prove particularly suitable for patients with CHD. Remote monitoring technologies, including wearable sensors and implantable cardiac devices, enable the continuous assessment of physical activity levels, arrhythmic events, and overall adherence to exercise prescription [52].

5. Special Needs Patient Population

5.1. Pulmonary Hypertension

In patients with pulmonary arterial hypertension (PAH) secondary to congenital heart disease (CHD), right ventricular (RV) afterload is chronically elevated. Initially, the right heart undergoes adaptive remodeling characterized by concentric hypertrophy to preserve systolic function. However, this compensatory mechanism may become maladaptive over time, resulting in progressive systolic dysfunction and RV dilation. In individuals with

Eisenmenger syndrome, this adaptive hypertrophic response may remain sustained into late adulthood.

In the previously implemented clinical practice, ET and cardiopulmonary rehabilitation were considered contraindicated in patients with pulmonary hypertension (PH), owing to concerns regarding patient safety, including the potential risk of sudden cardiac death, aggravation of pulmonary vascular remodeling, and progressive right ventricular dysfunction. Accordingly, patients with PH were routinely advised to abstain from physical activity.

While low-to moderate-intensity physical activity is generally well tolerated in patients with PH and has been shown to confer clinical benefits, high-intensity exercise may carry an elevated risk of adverse events, including hypotension due to reduced cardiac output, syncope, and sudden cardiac death. However, a meta-analysis by Zeng et al. reported a very low incidence of adverse events (~3.5%), with no major complications such as severe right heart failure, disease worsening, or death [53].

A meta-analysis of 9 randomized controlled trials (total number of 302 participants) demonstrated that ET significantly improved VO_2-peak (mean increase of approx. +2.79 $mL \cdot kg^{-1} \cdot min^{-1}$), anaerobic threshold (approx. +107 $mL \cdot min^{-1}$), and 6-min walk distance (6MWD) by an average of +46.7 m. In addition, both physical and mental scores in the SF-36 quality of life questionnaire improved significantly [54]. Systematic reviews confirm that physical training can reduce resting pulmonary artery systolic pressure (PASP), improve pulmonary perfusion, and enhance overall cardiopulmonary function [53]. Although it is relatively rare, some patients with PAH have exertional angina, resulting from compression of the left main coronary artery by a dilated pulmonary artery, such a phenomenon may be exacerbated during physical activity.

5.2. Desaturation

In individuals with cyanotic congenital heart disease (CHD), baseline arterial oxygen saturation may be markedly reduced, with significant desaturation occurring even during low-intensity activity. Those with right-to-left shunting or diminished pulmonary blood flow are particularly susceptible to desaturation during exercise. For patients with severe cyanosis, both exercise intensity and duration should therefore be guided by symptom limitation and subjective ratings of perceived exertion. In selected frail patients, a modest improvement in oxygen saturation may be achieved through supplemental oxygen, which can occasionally be considered as an adjunct during exercise testing or training [42].

5.3. Pathologies of the Aorta

Following the repair of a coarctation, the primary long-term concern is systemic hypertension. Patients may present with normotension at rest yet demonstrate a pronounced hypertensive response even to minimal physical exertion, underscoring the importance of careful monitoring of blood pressure and heart rate during exercise [29,42,55]. In individuals with repaired coarctation of the aorta, exercise testing is recommended to evaluate the hemodynamic response to physical stress. Based on the results, individuals with a significant hypertensive response to exercise may need to avoid activities with a high static load that can cause a sharp rise in blood pressure. Regular aerobic exercise is generally beneficial and encouraged to help manage resting blood pressure [55,56]. Patients presenting with significant aortic dilatation or obstructive lesions should be restricted to low-intensity ET until definitive surgical repair has been performed and formal medical clearance obtained [42]. Engagement in moderate- to high-intensity aerobic or resistance ET is theoretically associated with an increased risk of promoting aortic dilatation or, in rare instances, precipitating aortic dissection. Consequently, such forms of training are contraindicated in the presence of moderate or greater degrees of aortic dilatation, as well as in cases of documented aortic aneurysm or pseudoaneurysm [57].

5.4. Cardiac Implantable Electronic Devices

Following implantation, excessive upper extremity activity should be restricted for approximately 3–4 weeks to reduce the risk of lead displacement. In the longer term, patients with cardiac implantable devices are generally advised to avoid high-impact physical activities that may compromise device integrity. Endurance-based sports involving repetitive arm movements, such as long-distance swimming, can place mechanical stress on transvenous leads and may cause a predisposition to lead damage; such activities should therefore be approached with caution [42,58].

In individuals with ICDs, exercise intensity should be generally prescribed 10–15 beats per minute below the programmed detection threshold to minimize the risk of inappropriate shocks, unless advanced arrhythmia discrimination features are confirmed [59,60]. In patients with pacemakers, exercise generally poses fewer restrictions; however one should keep in mind that heart rate may be an unreliable marker of training intensity. Furthermore, individuals with complete heart block who rely on atrial-sensed, ventricular-paced modes may reach the device's upper tracking limit at higher exercise intensities, resulting in the abrupt loss of atrioventricular synchrony [42].

5.5. Fontan Circulation

Fontan circulation is characterized by the absence of a sub-pulmonary ventricle, resulting in passive pulmonary blood flow and inherently limited hemodynamic reserve. Such altered physiology constrains the ability to augment cardiac output during exertion, leading to reduced exercise tolerance [61]. Consequently, many Fontan patients adopt a sedentary lifestyle, which exacerbates skeletal muscle atrophy and further diminishes functional capacity [62]. According to European Society of Cardiology guidelines, moderate symptom-limited aerobic exercise is to be recommended to improve muscular strength and quality of life [5] A randomized trial combining aerobic and inspiratory muscle training increased peak VO_2 by ~23% ($27.0 \rightarrow 33.3$ $mL \cdot kg^{-1} \cdot min^{-1}$) versus usual care, with additional benefits from inspiratory training alone and no training-related serious events [62,63]. Multiple systematic reviews and meta-analyses confirm consistent improvements in exercise capacity, with signals for better ventilatory efficiency and quality of life, and very low adverse-event rates [64]. Leg-focused resistance programs have also proved beneficial for Fontan patients, as targeted strengthening of the lower limbs augments the skeletal muscle pump and venous return in the absence of a subpulmonary ventricle [50,65].

6. Conclusions

The clinical approach to physical activity in patients with congenital heart disease (CHD) has undergone a profound transformation over the past several decades and can be summarized in the following bullet points:

1. For the vast majority of patients, physical activity is not only safe but essential and should be strongly promoted.
2. Activity restrictions are now reserved for a very small subset of patients with specific high-risk conditions.
3. The contemporary role of the healthcare professional has expanded beyond simply permitting activity.
4. Physical activity counseling is considered an essential component of every patient interaction, regardless of whether the patient's clinical status warrants any restrictions.

5. The management of physical activity is a dynamic, lifelong process. The initial prescription is not static but must be subject to ongoing surveillance and adjustment

Historically, clinical practice was dominated by a paradigm of restriction, where patients were frequently advised to limit their physical activity. The overwhelming consensus is that a sedentary lifestyle poses a greater threat to the long-term health of most CHD patients than does participation in appropriate physical activity. The clinical imperative is therefore to safely guide patients toward achieving and maintaining an active life. It now involves actively counteracting the ingrained fear, parental overprotection, and physical deconditioning that resulted from previous medical guidance. Regular follow-up, including serial exercise testing, is essential for monitoring a patient's clinical trajectory. A spontaneous decline in a patient's habitual activity level should be treated as a potential early warning sign of clinical deterioration, prompting a thorough re-evaluation. Through a continuous cycle of evaluation, risk stratification, and prescription—all conducted within a framework of shared decision-making and empowering patient counseling—healthcare professionals can effectively and safely integrate physical activity as a core therapeutic modality, helping patients with congenital heart disease live longer, healthier, and more fulfilling lives.

Author Contributions: Conceptualization, D.F.-S., I.B. and A.B.-D.; Methodology, D.F.-S., I.B. and A.B.-D.; Validation, D.F.-S., I.B. and A.B.-D.; Formal Analysis, D.F.-S.; Investigation, D.F.-S.; Resources, D.F.-S., I.B. and A.B.-D.; Writing—Original Draft Preparation, D.F.-S.; Writing—Review & Editing, I.B. and A.B.-D.; Visualization, D.F.-S.; Supervision, A.B.-D. All authors have read and agreed to the published version of the manuscript.

Funding: This research received no external funding.

Conflicts of Interest: The authors declare no conflicts of interest.

Abbreviations

The following abbreviations are used in this manuscript:

6MWT	6-min walk test
AF	Atrial fibrillation
AFl	Atrial fluttering
Ao	Aorta
ccTGA	Congenitally corrected transposition of the great arteries
CHD	Congenital heart diseases
CMR	Cardiovascular magnetic resonance
CPET	Cardiopulmonary exercise test
CRF	Cardiorespiratory fitness
CT	Computed tomography
ECG	Electrocardiogram
EDA	End diastolic area
EDV	End diastolic volume
ET	Exercise training
FAC	Fractional area change
HITT	High-intensity interval training
HRR	Heart rate reserve
LV	Left ventricle
LVEDD	Left ventricular end diastolic diameter
LVEF	Left ventricular ejection fraction
LVESD	Left ventricular end systolic diameter
LVOT	Left ventricular outflow tract

NsVT	Non-sustained ventricular tachycardia
PAH	Pulmonary arterial hypertension
PASP	Pulmonary artery systolic pressure
PVC	Premature ventricular complex
RPE	Rate of perceived exertion
RV	Right ventricle
RVEDD	Right ventricular end diastolic diameter
RVOT	Right ventricular outflow tract
SPAP	Systolic pulmonary artery pressure
SpO_2	Oxygen saturation
TAPSE	Tricuspid annular plane systolic excursion
TRV	Tricuspid regurgitant velocity
VAT	Ventilatory anaerobic threshold
VE/VCO_2	Ventilation to carbon dioxide output
VO_2	Oxygen uptake
VT	Ventricular tachycardia

References

1. Van Der Linde, D.; Konings, E.E.M.; Slager, M.A.; Witsenburg, M.; Helbing, W.A.; Takkenberg, J.J.M.; Roos-Hesselink, J.W. Birth Prevalence of Congenital Heart Disease Worldwide. *J. Am. Coll. Cardiol.* **2011**, *58*, 2241–2247. [CrossRef]
2. Van Der Bom, T.; Bouma, B.J.; Meijboom, F.J.; Zwinderman, A.H.; Mulder, B.J.M. The Prevalence of Adult Congenital Heart Disease, Results from a Systematic Review and Evidence Based Calculation. *Am. Heart J.* **2012**, *164*, 568–575. [CrossRef] [PubMed]
3. Moons, P.; Marelli, A. Born to Age: When Adult Congenital Heart Disease Converges with Geroscience. *JACC Adv.* **2022**, *1*, 100012. [CrossRef]
4. Dellborg, M. Adult Congenital Heart Disease. *Circulation* **2024**, *149*, 1397–1399. [CrossRef]
5. Baumgartner, H.; De Backer, J.; Babu-Narayan, S.V.; Budts, W.; Chessa, M.; Diller, G.-P.; Lung, B.; Kluin, J.; Lang, I.M.; Meijboom, F.; et al. 2020 ESC Guidelines for the Management of Adult Congenital Heart Disease. *Eur. Heart J.* **2021**, *42*, 563–645. [CrossRef]
6. Reybrouck, T.; Mertens, L. Physical Performance and Physical Activity in Grown-up Congenital Heart Disease. *Eur. J. Cardiovasc. Prev. Rehabil.* **2005**, *12*, 498–502. [CrossRef] [PubMed]
7. Van Deutekom, A.W.; Lewandowski, A.J. Physical Activity Modification in Youth with Congenital Heart Disease: A Comprehensive Narrative Review. *Pediatr. Res.* **2021**, *89*, 1650–1658. [CrossRef]
8. Moons, P.; Deyk, K.V.; Dedroog, D.; Troost, E.; Budts, W. Prevalence of Cardiovascular Risk Factors in Adults with Congenital Heart Disease. *Eur. J. Cardiovasc. Prev. Rehabil.* **2006**, *13*, 612–616. [CrossRef] [PubMed]
9. Lin, Y.-S.; Liu, P.-H.; Wu, L.-S.; Chen, Y.-M.; Chang, C.-J.; Chu, P.-H. Major Adverse Cardiovascular Events in Adult Congenital Heart Disease: A Population-Based Follow-up Study from Taiwan. *BMC Cardiovasc. Disord.* **2014**, *14*, 38. [CrossRef]
10. Afilalo, J.; Therrien, J.; Pilote, L.; Ionescu-Ittu, R.; Martucci, G.; Marelli, A.J. Geriatric Congenital Heart Disease. *J. Am. Coll. Cardiol.* **2011**, *58*, 1509–1515. [CrossRef]
11. Zomer, A.C.; Vaartjes, I.; Uiterwaal, C.S.P.; Van Der Velde, E.T.; Sieswerda, G.-J.T.; Wajon, E.M.C.; Plomp, K.; Van Bergen, P.F.M.; Verheugt, C.L.; Krivka, E.; et al. Social Burden and Lifestyle in Adults with Congenital Heart Disease. *Am. J. Cardiol.* **2012**, *109*, 1657–1663. [CrossRef]
12. Lui, G.K.; Rogers, I.S.; Ding, V.Y.; Hedlin, H.K.; MacMillen, K.; Maron, D.J.; Sillman, C.; Romfh, A.; Dade, T.C.; Haeffele, C.; et al. Risk Estimates for Atherosclerotic Cardiovascular Disease in Adults with Congenital Heart Disease. *Am. J. Cardiol.* **2017**, *119*, 112–118. [CrossRef]
13. Tutarel, O. Acquired Heart Conditions in Adults with Congenital Heart Disease: A Growing Problem. *Heart* **2014**, *100*, 1317–1321. [CrossRef] [PubMed]
14. Franklin, B.A.; Lavie, C.J.; Squires, R.W.; Milani, R.V. Exercise-Based Cardiac Rehabilitation and Improvements in Cardiorespiratory Fitness: Implications Regarding Patient Benefit. *Mayo Clin. Proc.* **2013**, *88*, 431–437. [CrossRef] [PubMed]
15. Budts, W.; Borjesson, M.; Chessa, M.; Van Buuren, F.; Trigo Trindade, P.; Corrado, D.; Heidbuchel, H.; Webb, G.; Holm, J.; Papadakis, M. Physical Activity in Adolescents and Adults with Congenital Heart Defects: Individualized Exercise Prescription. *Eur. Heart J.* **2013**, *34*, 3669–3674. [CrossRef]
16. Galderisi, M.; Cosyns, B.; Edvardsen, T.; Cardim, N.; Delgado, V.; Di Salvo, G.; Donal, E.; Sade, L.E.; Ernande, L.; Garbi, M.; et al. Standardization of Adult Transthoracic Echocardiography Reporting in Agreement with Recent Chamber Quantification, Diastolic Function, and Heart Valve Disease Recommendations: An Expert Consensus Document of the European Association of Cardiovascular Imaging. *Eur. Heart J.-Cardiovasc. Imaging* **2017**, *18*, 1301–1310. [CrossRef] [PubMed]

17. Lang, R.M.; Badano, L.P.; Mor-Avi, V.; Afilalo, J.; Armstrong, A.; Ernande, L.; Flachskampf, F.A.; Foster, E.; Goldstein, S.A.; Kuznetsova, T.; et al. Recommendations for Cardiac Chamber Quantification by Echocardiography in Adults: An Update from the American Society of Echocardiography and the European Association of Cardiovascular Imaging. *Eur. Heart J. Cardiovasc. Imaging* **2015**, *16*, 233–271. [CrossRef]
18. Di Salvo, G.; Miller, O.; Babu Narayan, S.; Li, W.; Budts, W.; Valsangiacomo Buechel, E.R.; Frigiola, A.; Van Den Bosch, A.E.; Bonello, B.; Mertens, L.; et al. Imaging the Adult with Congenital Heart Disease: A Multimodality Imaging Approach—Position Paper from the EACVI. *Eur. Heart J.-Cardiovasc. Imaging* **2018**, *19*, 1077–1098. [CrossRef]
19. Budts, W.; Pieles, G.E.; Roos-Hesselink, J.W.; Sanz De La Garza, M.; D'Ascenzi, F.; Giannakoulas, G.; Müller, J.; Oberhoffer, R.; Ehringer-Schetitska, D.; Herceg-Cavrak, V.; et al. Recommendations for Participation in Competitive Sport in Adolescent and Adult Athletes with Congenital Heart Disease (CHD): Position Statement of the Sports Cardiology & Exercise Section of the European Association of Preventive Cardiology (EAPC), the European Society of Cardiology (ESC) Working Group on Adult Congenital Heart Disease and the Sports Cardiology, Physical Activity and Prevention Working Group of the Association for European Paediatric and Congenital Cardiology (AEPC). *Eur. Heart J.* **2020**, *41*, 4191–4199. [CrossRef]
20. Pelliccia, A.; Sharma, S.; Gati, S.; Bäck, M.; Börjesson, M.; Caselli, S.; Collet, J.-P.; Corrado, D.; Drezner, J.A.; Halle, M.; et al. 2020 ESC Guidelines on Sports Cardiology and Exercise in Patients with Cardiovascular Disease. *Eur. Heart J.* **2021**, *42*, 17–96. [CrossRef]
21. Khairy, P. Arrhythmias and Sudden Cardiac Death in Adult Congenital Heart Disease. In *Clinical Approach to Sudden Cardiac Death Syndromes*; Brugada, R., Ed.; Springer: London, UK, 2010; pp. 37–56, ISBN 978-1-84882-926-8.
22. Krieger, E.V.; Zeppenfeld, K.; DeWitt, E.S.; Duarte, V.E.; Egbe, A.C.; Haeffele, C.; Lin, K.Y.; Robinson, M.R.; Sillman, C.; Upadhyay, S.; et al. Arrhythmias in Repaired Tetralogy of Fallot: A Scientific Statement From the American Heart Association. *Circ. Arrhythmia Electrophysiol.* **2022**, *15*, e000084. [CrossRef]
23. Small, A.J.; Dai, M.; Halpern, D.G.; Tan, R.B. Updates in Arrhythmia Management in Adult Congenital Heart Disease. *J. Clin. Med.* **2024**, *13*, 4314. [CrossRef]
24. Cifra, B.; Cordina, R.L.; Gauthier, N.; Murphy, L.C.; Pham, T.D.; Veldtman, G.R.; Ward, K.; White, D.A.; Paridon, S.M.; Powell, A.W.; et al. Cardiopulmonary Exercise Test Interpretation Across the Lifespan in Congenital Heart Disease: A Scientific Statement From the American Heart Association. *JAHA* **2025**, *14*, e038200. [CrossRef]
25. Guglielmi, G.; Moscatelli, S.; Rocchetti, G.; Agostoni, P.; Chessa, M.; Mapelli, M. Cardiopulmonary Exercise Testing in Congenital Heart Disease: A Never-Ending Story from Paediatrics to Adult Life. *Children* **2025**, *12*, 1175. [CrossRef]
26. Inuzuka, R.; Diller, G.-P.; Borgia, F.; Benson, L.; Tay, E.L.W.; Alonso-Gonzalez, R.; Silva, M.; Charalambides, M.; Swan, L.; Dimopoulos, K.; et al. Comprehensive Use of Cardiopulmonary Exercise Testing Identifies Adults With Congenital Heart Disease at Increased Mortality Risk in the Medium Term. *Circulation* **2012**, *125*, 250–259. [CrossRef]
27. Giardini, A.; Specchia, S.; Tacy, T.A.; Coutsoumbas, G.; Gargiulo, G.; Donti, A.; Formigari, R.; Bonvicini, M.; Picchio, F.M. Usefulness of Cardiopulmonary Exercise to Predict Long-Term Prognosis in Adults with Repaired Tetralogy of Fallot. *Am. J. Cardiol.* **2007**, *99*, 1462–1467. [CrossRef]
28. Udholm, S.; Aldweib, N.; Hjortdal, V.E.; Veldtman, G.R. Prognostic Power of Cardiopulmonary Exercise Testing in Fontan Patients: A Systematic Review. *Open Heart* **2018**, *5*, e000812. [CrossRef]
29. Kempny, A.; Dimopoulos, K.; Uebing, A.; Moceri, P.; Swan, L.; Gatzoulis, M.A.; Diller, G.-P. Reference Values for Exercise Limitations among Adults with Congenital Heart Disease. Relation to Activities of Daily Life--Single Centre Experience and Review of Published Data. *Eur. Heart J.* **2012**, *33*, 1386–1396. [CrossRef] [PubMed]
30. Milani, J.G.P.O.; Milani, M.; Verboven, K.; Cipriano, G.; Hansen, D. Exercise Intensity Prescription in Cardiovascular Rehabilitation: Bridging the Gap between Best Evidence and Clinical Practice. *Front. Cardiovasc. Med.* **2024**, *11*, 1380639. [CrossRef] [PubMed]
31. Hansen, D.; Abreu, A.; Ambrosetti, M.; Cornelissen, V.; Gevaert, A.; Kemps, H.; Laukkanen, J.A.; Pedretti, R.; Simonenko, M.; Wilhelm, M.; et al. Exercise Intensity Assessment and Prescription in Cardiovascular Rehabilitation and beyond: Why and How: A Position Statement from the Secondary Prevention and Rehabilitation Section of the European Association of Preventive Cardiology. *Eur. J. Prev. Cardiol.* **2022**, *29*, 230–245. [CrossRef] [PubMed]
32. Koyak, Z.; Harris, L.; De Groot, J.R.; Silversides, C.K.; Oechslin, E.N.; Bouma, B.J.; Budts, W.; Zwinderman, A.H.; Van Gelder, I.C.; Mulder, B.J.M. Sudden Cardiac Death in Adult Congenital Heart Disease. *Circulation* **2012**, *126*, 1944–1954. [CrossRef]
33. Norozi, K.; Wessel, A.; Alpers, V.; Arnhold, J.O.; Binder, L.; Geyer, S.; Zoege, M.; Buchhorn, R. Chronotropic Incompetence in Adolescents and Adults with Congenital Heart Disease After Cardiac Surgery. *J. Card. Fail.* **2007**, *13*, 263–268. [CrossRef]
34. Gatzoulis, M.A.; Beghetti, M.; Landzberg, M.J.; Galiè, N. Pulmonary Arterial Hypertension Associated with Congenital Heart Disease: Recent Advances and Future Directions. *Int. J. Cardiol.* **2014**, *177*, 340–347. [CrossRef]
35. Miranda, W.R.; Aboulhosn, J.A.; Hagler, D.J. Catheterization in Adults with Congenital Heart Disease. *JACC Cardiovasc. Interv.* **2022**, *15*, 907–921. [CrossRef]
36. Jokinen, E. Coronary Artery Disease in Patients with Congenital Heart Defects. *J. Intern. Med.* **2020**, *288*, 383–389. [CrossRef]

37. Shah, S.S.; Mohanty, S.; Karande, T.; Maheshwari, S.; Kulkarni, S.; Saxena, A. Guidelines for Physical Activity in Children with Heart Disease. *Ann. Pediatr. Cardiol.* **2022**, *15*, 467–488. [CrossRef]
38. Takken, T.; Giardini, A.; Reybrouck, T.; Gewillig, M.; Hövels-Gürich, H.; Longmuir, P.; McCrindle, B.; Paridon, S.; Hager, A. Recommendations for Physical Activity, Recreation Sport, and Exercise Training in Paediatric Patients with Congenital Heart Disease: A Report from the Exercise, Basic & Translational Research Section of the European Association of Cardiovascular Prevention and Rehabilitation, the European Congenital Heart and Lung Exercise Group, and the Association for European Paediatric Cardiology. *Eur. J. Prev. Cardiol.* **2012**, *19*, 1034–1065. [CrossRef]
39. Piercy, K.L.; Troiano, R.P. Physical Activity Guidelines for Americans from the US Department of Health and Human Services. Cardiovascular Benefits and Recommendations. *Circ. Cardiovasc. Qual. Outcomes* **2018**, *11*, e005263. [CrossRef]
40. Longmuir, P.E.; Brothers, J.A.; De Ferranti, S.D.; Hayman, L.L.; Van Hare, G.F.; Matherne, G.P.; Davis, C.K.; Joy, E.A.; McCrindle, B.W. Promotion of Physical Activity for Children and Adults with Congenital Heart Disease: A Scientific Statement from the American Heart Association. *Circulation* **2013**, *127*, 2147–2159. [CrossRef]
41. Becker-Grünig, T.; Klose, H.; Ehlken, N.; Lichtblau, M.; Nagel, C.; Fischer, C.; Gorenflo, M.; Tiede, H.; Schranz, D.; Hager, A.; et al. Efficacy of Exercise Training in Pulmonary Arterial Hypertension Associated with Congenital Heart Disease. *Int. J. Cardiol.* **2013**, *168*, 375–381. [CrossRef]
42. Tran, D.; Maiorana, A.; Ayer, J.; Lubans, D.R.; Davis, G.M.; Celermajer, D.S.; d'Udekem, Y.; Cordina, R. Recommendations for Exercise in Adolescents and Adults with Congenital Heart Disease. *Prog. Cardiovasc. Dis.* **2020**, *63*, 350–366. [CrossRef]
43. Opocher, F.; Varnier, M.; Sanders, S.P.; Tosoni, A.; Zaccaria, M.; Stellin, G.; Milanesi, O. Effects of Aerobic Exercise Training in Children after the Fontan Operation. *Am. J. Cardiol.* **2005**, *95*, 150–152. [CrossRef]
44. Bhasipol, A.; Sanjaroensuttikul, N.; Pornsuriyasak, P.; Yamwong, S.; Tangcharoen, T. Efficiency of the Home Cardiac Rehabilitation Program for Adults with Complex Congenital Heart Disease. *Congenit. Heart Dis.* **2018**, *13*, 952–958. [CrossRef]
45. Rocha Conceição, L.S.; Gauthier, N.; Andrade Guimarães, A.L.; Gois, C.O.; Oliveira, I.K.; Souza, D.S.; Carvalho, V.O. High-Intensity Interval Training in Adults with Congenital Heart Disease: A Systematic Review. *Heart Lung Circ.* **2025**, *34*, 16–24. [CrossRef]
46. Novaković, M.; Prokšelj, K.; Rajkovič, U.; Vižintin Cuderman, T.; Janša Trontelj, K.; Fras, Z.; Jug, B. Exercise Training in Adults with Repaired Tetralogy of Fallot: A Randomized Controlled Pilot Study of Continuous versus Interval Training. *Int. J. Cardiol.* **2018**, *255*, 37–44. [CrossRef]
47. Hao, K.; Wadey, C.A.; Barker, A.R.; Williams, C.A. The Effect of Strength Training Interventions on People with Congenital Heart Disease: A Systematic Review. *Open Heart* **2025**, *12*, e003091. [CrossRef]
48. Garber, C.E.; Blissmer, B.; Deschenes, M.R.; Franklin, B.A.; Lamonte, M.J.; Lee, I.-M.; Nieman, D.C.; Swain, D.P. Quantity and Quality of Exercise for Developing and Maintaining Cardiorespiratory, Musculoskeletal, and Neuromotor Fitness in Apparently Healthy Adults: Guidance for Prescribing Exercise. *Med. Sci. Sports Exerc.* **2011**, *43*, 1334–1359. [CrossRef]
49. Cordina, R.L.; O'Meagher, S.; Karmali, A.; Rae, C.L.; Liess, C.; Kemp, G.J.; Puranik, R.; Singh, N.; Celermajer, D.S. Resistance Training Improves Cardiac Output, Exercise Capacity and Tolerance to Positive Airway Pressure in Fontan Physiology. *Int. J. Cardiol.* **2013**, *168*, 780–788. [CrossRef]
50. Avitabile, C.M.; Goldberg, D.J.; Leonard, M.B.; Wei, Z.A.; Tang, E.; Paridon, S.M.; Yoganathan, A.P.; Fogel, M.A.; Whitehead, K.K. Leg Lean Mass Correlates with Exercise Systemic Output in Young Fontan Patients. *Heart* **2018**, *104*, 680–684. [CrossRef]
51. Vanhees, L.; Stevens, A. Exercise Intensity: A Matter of Measuring or of Talking? *J. Cardiopulm. Rehabil.* **2006**, *26*, 78–79. [CrossRef]
52. Matteucci, A.; Bonanni, M.; Centioni, M.; Zanin, F.; Geuna, F.; Massaro, G.; Sangiorgi, G. Home Management of Heart Failure and Arrhythmias in Patients with Cardiac Devices during Pandemic. *J. Clin. Med.* **2021**, *10*, 1618. [CrossRef]
53. Zeng, X.; Chen, H.; Ruan, H.; Ye, X.; Li, J.; Hong, C. Effectiveness and Safety of Exercise Training and Rehabilitation in Pulmonary Hypertension: A Systematic Review and Meta-Analysis. *J. Thorac. Dis.* **2020**, *12*, 2691–2705. [CrossRef]
54. Albanaqi, A.L.; Rahimi, G.R.M.; Smart, N.A. Exercise Training for Pulmonary Hypertension: A Systematic Review and Meta-Analysis of Randomized Controlled Trials. *Biol. Res. Nurs.* **2021**, *23*, 442–454. [CrossRef]
55. Stout, K.K.; Daniels, C.J.; Aboulhosn, J.A.; Bozkurt, B.; Broberg, C.S.; Colman, J.M.; Crumb, S.R.; Dearani, J.A.; Fuller, S.; Gurvitz, M.; et al. 2018 AHA/ACC Guideline for the Management of Adults With Congenital Heart Disease: A Report of the American College of Cardiology/American Heart Association Task Force on Clinical Practice Guidelines. *Circulation* **2019**, *139*, e637–e697. [CrossRef]
56. Clarkson, P.M.; Nicholson, M.R.; Barratt-Boyes, B.G.; Neutze, J.M.; Whitlock, R.M. Results after Repair of Coarctation of the Aorta beyond Infancy: A 10 to 28 Year Follow-up with Particular Reference to Late Systemic Hypertension. *Am. J. Cardiol.* **1983**, *51*, 1481–1488. [CrossRef]
57. Gati, S.; Malhotra, A.; Sharma, S. Exercise Recommendations in Patients with Valvular Heart Disease. *Heart* **2019**, *105*, 106–110. [CrossRef]
58. Kiuchi, V. Lifestyle Advice for Patients with ICDs: Physical Activity—What Is Healthy and What Is Contraindicated. *e-J. Cardiol. Pract.* **2019**, *17*.

59. Fletcher, G.F.; Ades, P.A.; Kligfield, P.; Arena, R.; Balady, G.J.; Bittner, V.A.; Coke, L.A.; Fleg, J.L.; Forman, D.E.; Gerber, T.C.; et al. Exercise Standards for Testing and Training: A Scientific Statement From the American Heart Association. *Circulation* **2013**, *128*, 873–934. [CrossRef]
60. Steinhaus, D.A.; Lubitz, S.A.; Noseworthy, P.A.; Kramer, D.B. Exercise Interventions in Patients With Implantable Cardioverter-Defibrillators and Cardiac Resynchronization Therapy: A Systematic Review and Meta-Analysis. *J. Cardiopulm. Rehabil. Prev.* **2019**, *39*, 308–317. [CrossRef]
61. Gewillig, M. The Fontan Circulation. *Heart* **2005**, *91*, 839–846. [CrossRef]
62. Ven, L.V.D.; Félix, A.C.; Suarez, J.; Dias, J.; Pinto, F.F.; Laranjo, S. Cardiac Rehabilitation for Fontan Circulation Patients: A Systematic Review, and Meta-Analysis. *Medicina* **2024**, *60*, 1817. [CrossRef] [PubMed]
63. Turquetto, A.L.R.; Dos Santos, M.R.; Agostinho, D.R.; Sayegh, A.L.C.; De Souza, F.R.; Amato, L.P.; Barnabe, M.S.R.; De Oliveira, P.A.; Liberato, G.; Binotto, M.A.; et al. Aerobic Exercise and Inspiratory Muscle Training Increase Functional Capacity in Patients with Univentricular Physiology after Fontan Operation: A Randomized Controlled Trial. *Int. J. Cardiol.* **2021**, *330*, 50–58. [CrossRef] [PubMed]
64. Choi, H.J.; Kim, S.-J.; Lee, D.W.; Gwon, S.H.; Son, N.-H.; Cho, M.J.; Oh, K.J.; Lee, J.S.; Na, J.Y.; Seol, J.H. Effects of Exercise Training in Patients with Fontan Circulation: A Systematic Review and Meta-Analysis. *Korean Circ. J.* **2025**, *55*, e63. [CrossRef] [PubMed]
65. Scheffers, L.E.; Helbing, W.A.; Pereira, T.; Utens, E.M.W.J.; Dulfer, K.; Hirsch, A.; Koopman, L.P.; Van Den Berg, L.E. Leg-Focused High-Weight Resistance Training Improves Ventricular Stroke Volume, Exercise Capacity and Strength in Young Patients with a Fontan Circulation. *Eur. J. Prev. Cardiol.* **2024**, *31*, 389–399. [CrossRef]

Journal of
Clinical Medicine

MDPI

Article

Implementation of a Hybrid Cardiac Rehabilitation and Symptom Scoring System in Patients with Inappropriate or Postural Sinus Tachycardia Referred for Sinus Node Sparing Hybrid Ablation

Marta Kornaszewska [1,2,*], Aleksandra Wilczek-Banc [3], Anna Ratajska [4,5], Ewa Piotrowicz [6], Bartosz Szkaradek [7], Mariusz Kowalewski [1,8,9,10], Piotr Suwalski [11], Natalia Ogorzelec [1], Antoni Wileczek [12], Magdalena Zając [13], Michał Pastyrzak [14,15] and Sebastian Stec [1,7,16]

1 Department of Cardiac Surgery and Transplantology, National Medical Institute of the Ministry of Interior and Administration, 02-507 Warsaw, Poland; natalia.ogorzelec@pimmswia.gov.pl (N.O.); smstec@wp.pl (S.S.)
2 Private Cardiology Practice, 33-394 Kleczany, Poland
3 Cardiac Rehabilitation Hospital, 38-481 Rymanów Zdrój, Poland; olabanc@gmail.com
4 Psychological Therapeutic and Research Center, Dr Jan Biziel University Hospital No. 2, 85-168 Bydgoszcz, Poland; aniarat@wp.pl
5 Department of Humanization Medicine and Sexology, Collegium Medicum, University of Zielona Góra, 65-048 Zielona Góra, Poland
6 Telecardiology Center National Institute of Cardiology, 04-628 Warsaw, Poland; epiotrowicz@ikard.pl
7 Institute for Cardiovascular Science, CardioNeuroLab, CardioMedicum, 30-002 Cracow, Poland; fnszkaradekbartosz@gmail.com
8 Cardio-Thoracic Surgery Department, Heart and Vascular Centre, Maastricht University Medical Centre, 6229 HX Maastricht, The Netherlands
9 Department for the Treatment and Study of Cardiothoracic Diseases and Cardiothoracic Transplantation, IRCCS-ISMETT, 90127 Palermo, Italy
10 Thoracic Research Center, Collegium Medicum, Nicolaus Copernicus University, Innovative Medical Forum, 85-067 Bydgoszcz, Poland
11 National Medical Institute of the Ministry of Interior and Administration, Centre of Postgraduate Medical Education, 02-507 Warsaw, Poland; suwalski.piotr@gmail.com
12 Panaceum-Med., Przemyska 24, 38-500 Sanok, Poland
13 Department of Special Pedagogy and Speech Therapy, Faculty of Pedagogy, Kazimierz Wielki University, 85-064 Bydgoszcz, Poland; nzozermed@wp.pl
14 Faculty of Physiotherapy, Jan Grodek State University in Sanok, 38-500 Sanok, Poland; michalpastyrzak@gmail.com
15 Private Physiotherapy Michał Pastyrzak, 38-500 Sanok, Poland
16 Elmedica EP-Network SKA, 26-110 Skarżysko-Kamienna, Poland
* Correspondence: mkornaszewska@gmail.com; Tel.: +48-793298288

Abstract: Background/Objectives: Patients with inappropriate sinus tachycardia (IST) and postural orthostatic tachycardia syndrome (POTS) exhibit complex clinical profiles due to autonomic dysfunction. While sinus node sparing (SNS) hybrid ablation is emerging as a promising therapy, there are no established guidelines worldwide for post-procedure patient management and care is mainly based on telemonitoring. In contrast, our hybrid cardiac rehabilitation (HCR) program integrates inpatient care and home-based telerehabilitation. We aim to evaluate the implementation of the HCR program, patient acceptance and adherence, and the effectiveness of the Malmö POTS scoring system in monitoring disease progression and rehabilitation outcomes. **Methods**: Patients underwent a personalized HCR program after SNS. The program included early mobilization, psychological support, respiratory therapy, and structured exercise. Clinical outcomes were assessed using symptom burden (Malmö POTS score), ECG parameters, exercise duration, perceived exertion, and rehabilitation adherence. **Results:** All patients completed the inpatient phase, and 87% completed the home-based phase. In the early postoperative period, pericarditis, anemia, and benign rhythm disturbances were mild and self-limiting. The Malmö POTS score decreased from 65.3 to 25.7. Lower perceived exertion early in the program correlated with clinical improvement. At the 2-month follow-up, 81% of patients no longer met the clinical criteria for IST/POTS without the use of medications. The program was evaluated as safe, feasible, and well-tolerated, with high patient satisfaction. **Conclusions**: A well-organized hybrid cardiac rehabilitation program after SNS is feasible, safe, and well-tolerated in IST/POTS patients. The Malmö POTS score may support outcome monitoring. The integration of individualized training and telemedicine represents a promising development for patients post-SNS ablation. While this study demonstrates feasibility and potential benefits, further controlled studies are needed to evaluate its impact on long-term recovery and symptom control.

Keywords: inappropriate sinus tachycardia; postural orthostatic tachycardia syndrome; sinus node-sparing hybrid ablation; hybrid cardiac rehabilitation; implementation

1. Introduction

Patients with inappropriate sinus tachycardia (IST) and postural orthostatic tachycardia syndrome (POTS) often present with complex clinical profiles [1,2], including multiple phenotypes and multi-organ abnormalities associated with cardiovascular autonomic dysfunction (CVAD). Therefore, their management should include comprehensive and long-term rehabilitation tailored to the patient's capacity, particularly in individuals with orthostatic intolerance [3]. Pharmacological treatment is primarily based on ivabradine [4] and/or beta-blockers administered at optimized doses [2,5]. Additional recommendations include a high-salt diet (6–10 g/day) and increased fluid intake (2.5–3 L/day); using compression garments (covering large venous reservoirs in the lower limbs and the pelvic region); consuming small, low-carbohydrate meals; avoiding prolonged bed rest; performing counter-maneuvers to prevent syncope (e.g., leg crossing and muscle tensing); avoiding caffeine, alcohol, and excessive heat; and strengthening psychological and social support [6]. Patients with severe, pharmacologically resistant symptoms of IST/POTS require advanced diagnostic tools, such as standardized cardiovascular autonomic testing (CAT) and electrophysiological study (EPS), for accurate differential diagnosis and qualification for further treatment. Until recently, only patients with IST were referred for percutaneous catheter ablation (modification or complete ablation of the sinus node). According to the SUSRUTA registry, this procedure was associated with a 100% failure rate, a high risk of complications (e.g., phrenic nerve injury and superior vena cava stenosis), and the need for urgent or delayed pacemaker implantation in as many as 50% of patients in long-term follow-up [7]. Over the past decade, sinus node sparing (SNS) hybrid ablation has emerged as a promising alternative for IST, POTS, and overlapping IST/POTS syndromes [8]. Early outcomes are encouraging, demonstrating superior long-term efficacy and safety compared to conventional non-hybrid approaches. SNS is currently under global evaluation in the HEAL-IST trial and registry [9,10]. To date, no global guidelines, standardized rehabilitation programs, or routine care protocols have been established for this specific patient group. The approach to post-SNS in most countries is telemonitoring and telecare. In Belgium, for instance, patients undergo implantation of an Implantable Loop Recorder (ILR), followed by phone consultations and outpatient clinical check-ups [8,9]. Our approach went further by developing a hybrid cardiac rehabilitation (HCR) program that integrates both inpatient and home-based telerehabilitation. This study aims to evaluate the implementation, patient acceptance, and adherence to the HCR program and to assess the effectiveness of the Malmö POTS scoring system in monitoring disease progression and rehabilitation outcomes [11].

2. Materials and Methods

2.1. Patient Population

This study included consecutive patients who underwent SNS between September 2023 and December 2024 at the Department of Cardiac Surgery and Transplantology, National Medical Institute of the Ministry of the Interior and Administration in Warsaw. All participants had a confirmed diagnosis of IST or POTS. According to the 2015 ACC/AHA/HRS expert consensus statement [12] and the 2019 ESC guidelines [13], for IST, individuals presented with a resting sinus rhythm heart rate (HR) >100 bpm, a mean 24-h HR >90 bpm, and an excessive sinus rate response to minimal physical exertion; for POTS, subjects exhibited a sustained HR increase of $\geq$30 bpm (or $\geq$40 bpm in individuals under 19 years of age) within 10 min of standing, in the absence of orthostatic hypotension, and with chronic symptoms of orthostatic intolerance lasting $\geq$6 months. Patients were eligible if, in accordance with the definition, their symptoms persisted despite at least six months of optimized non-pharmacological treatment and if ineffectiveness or intolerance of at least two medications (e.g., beta-blockers, ivabradine, or their combination) was documented. In all cases, an electrophysiological study (EPS) was performed before SNS.

2.2. Study Protocol

This study was approved by the University of Rzeszow's Ethics Committee (decision number 5/4/2017-RARE-A-CAREgistry) and adhered to the Declaration of Helsinki. All participants gave their written informed consent. This study was designed as a prospective observational analysis in which patients underwent the SNS procedure. Immediately after the intervention, during hospitalization in the cardiac surgery department, early mobilization and clinical assessment were carried out. After discharge (typically on postoperative day 3), patients were referred to a specialized cardiac rehabilitation center for a 21-day inpatient rehabilitation program. At the beginning of this stage, a comprehensive clinical assessment was performed. Additional tests included complete blood count, C-reactive protein measurement, 24-h three-lead Holter ECG monitoring, transthoracic echocardiography, and ultrasound examination of the pleural cavities. Exercise training was conducted according to the FITT principle (Figure 1), determining the exercise dose in terms of frequency, intensity, time, and type. After 7 days, a 6-min walk test (6MWT) was performed, based on which patients were further qualified for training on a stationary cycle ergometer. The symptoms were assessed and monitored using the Malmö POTS score questionnaire system. In the next phase, patients participated in a 35-day home-based telerehabilitation based on Nordic walking, delivered via a hybrid smartphone platform. Before each session, patients measured their body weight, blood pressure, and oxygen saturation, performed a self-recorded ECG, and completed a symptom questionnaire. Different durations and tailored training were used. Sessions were ECG-monitored in real time to continuously assess heart rhythm and detect potential abnormalities that could occur after the procedure. After training, patients measured oxygen saturation and reported perceived exertion according to the modified Borg CR10 Category Ratio scale (0–10) (mBorg CR10). All data were automatically transmitted to the IT platform through a dedicated mobile application. Based on all collected measurements, together with the patient's clinical condition and reported well-being, the supervising medical team individually adjusted the type and intensity of training. Sessions were delivered in either continuous or interval formats, depending on the patient's exercise capacity and tolerance.

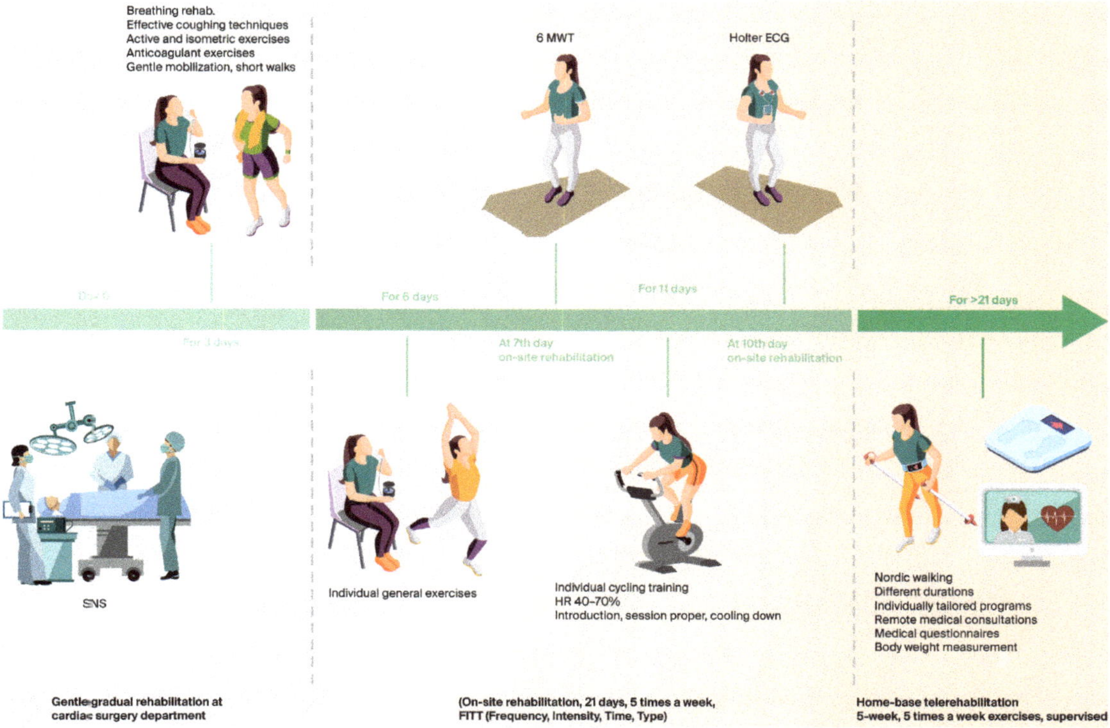

Figure 1. Timeline of the HCR protocol following SNS.

2.3. SNS Procedure

SNS was performed in all patients using the single-stage hybrid approach in accordance with previous reports and the HEAL-IST protocol [9]. In short, a multidisciplinary team performed the ablation, with a cardiac surgeon accessing the heart via a minimally invasive right thoracoscopic intercostal approach and an electrophysiologist using a femoral or left jugular venous route. High-density 3D mapping of the right atrium and activation patterns during sinus rhythm (EnSite NavX/Precision™, Abbott St. Paul, MN, USA) was conducted before and after surgery. A bipolar bidirectional RF clamp (AtriCure EMR2) was used to isolate the superior and inferior vena cava at their junctions with the right atrium. Endocardial mapping and pacing maneuvers were performed to confirm conduction block, and additional endocardial ablation was applied at the operator's discretion. Gentle, gradual mobilization as part of early recovery was initiated as early as the first postoperative day. After 3 days, participants were discharged with prophylactic ibuprofen, colchicine, and compressive stocks [14].

2.4. Program Protocol of Inpatient Rehabilitation

Inpatient rehabilitation based on the FITT principle was carried out under individual supervision. Exercise intensity was adjusted to the clinical condition and functional capacity of each patient [15,16]. The training process was divided into three stages: warm-up, main training, and cool-down [17]. The program began with gentle mobilization and breathing exercises, gradually progressing to general fitness exercises and interval endurance training on a stationary mini-cycle [16]. After seven days, the exercise capacity of stable patients was assessed using the 6MWT. In accordance with standard procedures, the test was performed between 10am and 12pm after the individuals had taken their regular medications. Markers were placed every 25 m, and patients performed a 6-min shuttle walk test. Subsequently, training sessions were conducted on a cycle ergometer, with individually adjusted workloads. The training heart rate was determined using the heart rate reserve method, which involves adding a specified percentage of the difference between maximal and resting heart rates to the resting heart rate, aiming to reach 40–70% of the heart rate reserve [16].

The program encompassed all aspects of cardiac rehabilitation care offered to patients, such as physical training, psychological support (including group and individual therapy), health education (lifestyle changes, nutrition, and physical activity), autogenic training, and individualized recommendations for physiotherapy. The primary goal was to optimize clinical status, improve physical fitness, prevent deconditioning, and restore functional independence.

2.5. Program Protocol of Home-Based Telerehabilitation

In the next stage, participants were referred to a telerehabilitation program based on a hybrid multi-recorder smartphone platform (DrEryk Kardio, Krakow, Poland). All sessions were monitored in real time by qualified medical personnel, enabling observation of the exercise course and immediate intervention in the event of symptoms. Telerehabilitation was implemented in the form of walking training via a smartphone platform, conducted as either continuous or interval walking (Nordic walking) [18,19]. Before each training session, the patient independently measured their blood pressure, body weight, and oxygen saturation; recorded an ECG using a wearable device; and completed a short pre-training questionnaire with the following questions: How are you feeling today? Have you taken all your medications? Do you have any symptoms of a cold or infection? All data were automatically transmitted to the telemedicine platform. The exclusion criteria for training were as follows: systolic blood pressure below 90 mmHg or above 160 mmHg, diastolic blood pressure below 50 mmHg or above 110 mmHg, an abnormal ECG recording (resting heart rate above 120 bpm, presence of conduction blocks, or arrhythmia), and feeling unwell or having symptoms of a cold. Continuous training sessions began with a 3- to 5-min warm-up and ended with a 5- to 10-min cool-down period (Figure 2a). In the interval training protocol, each session included alternating 5-min exercise and 5-min rest phases [17] (Figure 2b). All exercise phases were supervised by a programmed monitoring and control system capable of scheduling exercise intervals and transmitting ECG data [19] (Figure 3). Training was interrupted if HR fell outside the predefined range for each stage (80–120 and 80–140 bpm for continuous and interval training, respectively), or if the patient experienced malaise or alarming symptoms—in such cases, medical staff immediately contacted the subject. At the end of each session, the patient assessed the exertion performed using the mBorg CR10 and again measured oxygen saturation. These data were used to adjust the intensity of subsequent training sessions. The target exercise intensity was set at an mBorg CR10 value of 3, corresponding to moderate exertion. It is worth noting that, throughout the rehabilitation process, patients had the opportunity to participate in remote consultations with an electrophysiologist and a psychologist [20].

2.6. Clinical Assessment

On the second day of inpatient rehabilitation, echocardiographic examination and ultrasound of the pleural cavities were performed using a Philips Affinity 50G device. On the tenth day, a 24-h Holter ECG recording was obtained using a digital recorder (model DR 180+). To quantitatively assess symptom severity, the Malmö POTS scoring system questionnaire was used [10,11]. This questionnaire evaluates 12 of the most commonly reported symptoms, with a score from 0 (no symptom) to 10 (very severe symptom), yielding a total score range from 0 to 120 points. ECG monitoring and the active standing test were performed two months after completing the HCR program. The criteria for HCR effectiveness included both a reduction in the Malmö POTS score and the resolution of the clinical criteria for IST and POTS without pharmacotherapy. As the minimal clinically important change for the Malmö POTS scale has not yet been established, an improvement was defined as a score reduced below the validated diagnostic threshold of 42 points.

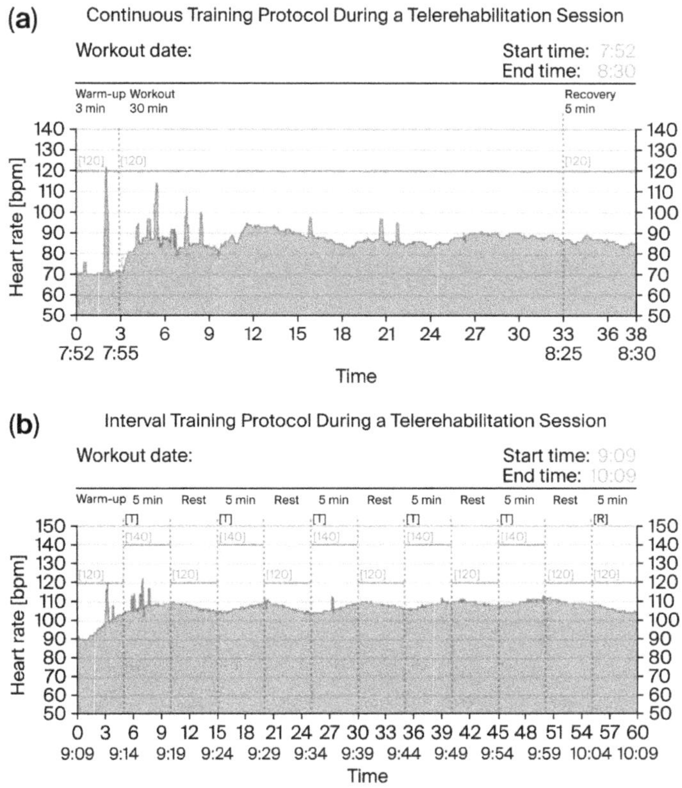

Figure 2. (**a**) Continuous training protocol of telerehabilitation session: commenced with a 3- to 5-min warm-up period, which was followed by 30 min of continuous exercise (target HR range 80–120 bpm), finishing with 5-min recovery period. Gray area—measured heart rate; colored horizontal lines—upper and lower HR limits (**b**) Interval training protocol during a telerehabilitation session: included alternating periods of 5-min exercises (target HR range: 80–140 bpm) and resting phases every other minute for the same duration. Session of 5 min exercise and 5 min rest phases, with the warm-up before, and cool-down following this interval session. Gray area—measured heart rate; colored horizontal lines—upper and lower HR margins.

2.7. Psychological Support

Patients received comprehensive psychological care before the procedure, along with continuous access to remote consultations throughout the entire rehabilitation process [20].

2.8. Statistical Analysis

Statistical analysis of the collected data was limited to descriptive statistics, including frequency distributions (expressed as percentages), mean values, standard deviation, and confidence intervals. No formal hypothesis testing was conducted. All calculations were performed using Statistica, version 13.0 (TIBCO Software Inc., 2623 Camino Ramon Suite 200, San Ramon, CA, USA).

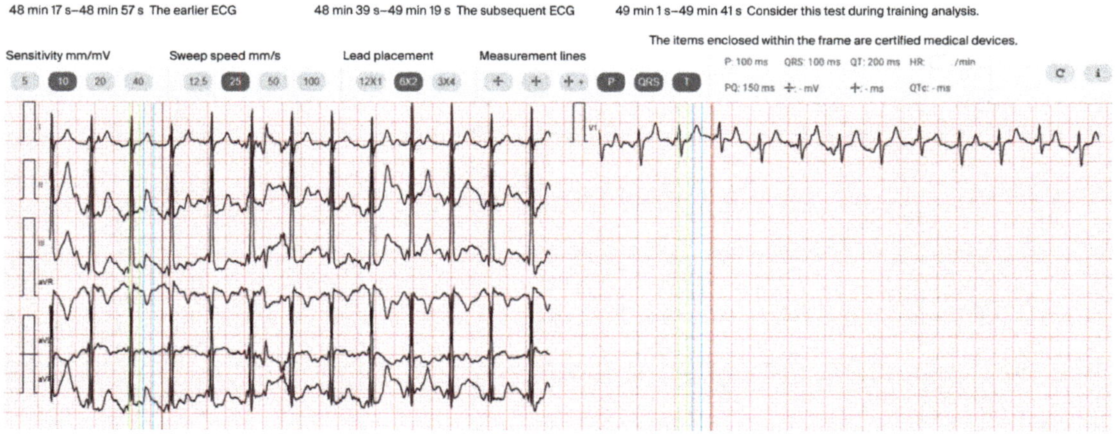

Figure 3. Continuous ECG monitoring performed with real-time data transmission to the online platform. Example of 49 min exercise recording showing continuous sinus rhythm at 136 bpm during training. The training data observed in real time is very high-quality and accurate, thus enabling precise patient monitoring and ensuring safety during training.

3. Results

During the EPS performed before SNS, slow–fast atrioventricular nodal reentrant tachycardia (AVNRT) ablation was carried out in seven cases (44%). Subsequently, SNS was successfully performed in all patients (100%) without significant early complications. Already on the first day of hospitalization, gentle and gradual mobilization was initiated, consisting of simple body weight exercises combined with stretching, breathing training, and strengthening exercises for small muscle groups. Within three days after the procedure, all patients were discharged from the hospital.

3.1. Implementation of Inpatient Rehabilitation and Early Clinical Events

All of the cohort (100%) finished inpatient rehabilitation that lasted 17.8 $\pm$ 4.2 days (mean $\pm$ STD). In the early postoperative period during inpatient rehabilitation, mild and transient symptoms of dyspnea and low exercise tolerance were observed in 10 out of 16 individuals (62%). In this group, unilateral and bilateral pleural effusions were present in five (50%) and three (30%) cases, respectively. Transient postcardiotomy syndrome was diagnosed in 9 out of 16 patients (44%) despite prophylactic colchicine administration in all cases (100%). The condition was self-limiting and did not lead to serious complications. Mild anemia (hemoglobin between 10 and 12 g/dL) was noted in eight cases (50%). Junctional accelerated rhythm and wandering atrial pacemakers were also observed in eight individuals (50%). Transient but echocardiographically significant tricuspid regurgitation (TR) was found in three patients (19%), including one case of severe TR (6%). Chest pain was reported by five cases (31%), with three individuals (19%) requiring additional consultations in the emergency department (emergency stay) due to the severity of symptoms; among them, two patients experienced panic attacks, and one reported chest pain caused by pleural effusion (Figure 4).

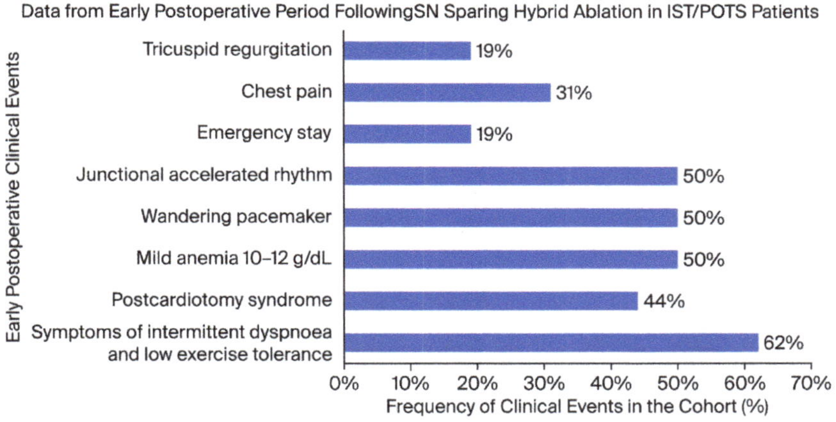

Figure 4. Frequency of early postoperative clinical events in a cohort of patients with IST/POTS undergoing sinus node sparing hybrid ablation. Data are presented as the percentage of patients in whom each of the described events was observed during the inpatient rehabilitation period. Reported events included tricuspid regurgitation, chest pain, unplanned emergency stay, junctional accelerated rhythm, wandering pacemaker, mild anemia (hemoglobin 10–12 g/dL), postcardiotomy syndrome, and intermittent dyspnea with low exercise tolerance. All conditions were self-limiting and did not result in serious complications.

3.2. *Efficacy of Inpatient Rehabilitation*

In the second week of rehabilitation, all patients (100%) underwent 24-h ECG monitoring using the Holter method. In the analyzed group, the average HR was 77.0 ± 18.5 bpm (CI + 95% 67.22–86.91). The mean minimum HR was 58.2 ± 17.5 bpm (CI + 95% 48.88–67.49), while the mean maximum HR reached 106.6 ± 17.5 bpm (CI + 95% 96.36–114.76). Particular attention was given to reducing the average HR below 90 bpm, which was a key therapeutic goal. This target was achieved in 10 cases (62%). While not a primary outcome, achieving average HR control may indicate favorable physiological adaptation during rehabilitation.

3.3. *Implementation and Acceptance of the Home-Based Telerehabilitation*

Home-based telerehabilitation was implemented immediately after the inpatient phase in 14 individuals (87%). All participants accepted the standard guidelines for the home-based stage, which included Nordic walking training. The treatment and rehabilitation program was supervised by a highly qualified cardiologist. Throughout the study, patients also had the opportunity to consult their physician via phone or email at any time.

3.4. *Adherence to Home-Based Telerehabilitation*

The average number of planned training sessions was 20.14 ± 10.1 meetings (mean ± STD). Patients finished about an average of 14.8 ± 8.71 sessions, with dropout rates for personal issues and medical causes only amounting to 0.64 ± 1.08 and 0.28 ± 0.47 sessions, respectively. The number of sessions missed was an average of 5.28 ± 5.6.

During the first training session, participants with higher systolic blood pressure at baseline exercised for a shorter duration and achieved lower peak heart rates. Conversely, those with a higher resting heart rate tended to train longer, reach higher HR values during exercise, and achieve better post-exercise oxygen saturation. This may suggest that a higher baseline HR is associated with better early exercise tolerance, whereas elevated blood pressure may limit initial physical capacity. No relationship was observed between these baseline values and perceived exertion on the mBorg CR10 scores. Interestingly, already in the first week, those who ultimately achieved clinical improvement often rated their sessions as less demanding and reported lower mBorg CR10 scores in sessions 3 and 6. This may suggest that an early subjective perception of exertion could be, to some extent, related to later clinical outcomes. Overall, mBorg CR10 scores were similar regardless of the type of training.

3.5. Clinical Assessment

A noticeable improvement in reported symptoms was observed over the course of the study. The mean Malmö POTS score decreased from 65.3 before the SNS procedure to 25.7 after completing rehabilitation. At the two-month follow-up, normalized Malmö POTS scores and resolved clinical diagnostic criteria for IST and POTS were recorded in 13 individuals (81%) without pharmacotherapy (confirmed via ECG monitoring and the active standing test) [21,22].

3.6. Psychological Support

Individual psychological consultations were conducted before and/or after the SNS hybrid ablation procedure. During pre-surgery consultations, patients presented their previous history of symptom management and psychological adaptation to the disease dynamics and narrated their psychosocial functioning (partner and social relationships, work, and emotions). We focused on preparing the patients and their families for upcoming surgery. We mainly worked on anxiety, managing the emotions of patients and their closest ones, and communication issues within the family. The postoperative period is worth dividing into immediate (up to one month), short (up to six months), and longer (more than six months) periods. Immediately after the operation, patients experienced various emotions: joy that their surgery had been successful, anxiety about what would happen next, and fear of pain. The dynamics and intensity of emotions were high. In the short postoperative period, patients achieved initial emotional stabilization; cognitive–behavioral work was necessary for some of them. Usually, pain was managed as the patient had the necessary knowledge and skills. Sometimes, there was fear of symptoms or illness returning. Simultaneously, they felt the willingness and fear of returning to their daily routine, normal life, and work. Patients reported a sense of inner change and a need to redefine their personal identities. As such, the field of psychotherapeutic work emerged. In the distant postoperative period, the psychological adaptation of patients to the changing situation and maintaining a balance between challenges to their new abilities (including physical), anxiety, and family dynamics requires attention. These psychological experiences may have influenced how patients engaged in exercise and perceived their symptoms, which in turn could have contributed to the improvement observed in the Malmö POTS score.

4. Discussion

Our observational study is the first to show that the HCR model—combining inpatient rehabilitation with home-based telerehabilitation—is feasible, safe, and well-tolerated by patients with IST and POTS undergoing SNS. Upon completing the program, the vast majority of participants no longer met the diagnostic criteria for IST/POTS [23]. These findings are consistent with current perspectives presented by Taylor and Blakemore (2025) [24], who emphasize the role of home-based cardiac rehabilitation in improving accessibility and adherence. While these authors note that some meta-analyses indicate slightly greater effects with inpatient rehabilitation, they also point out that more recent data suggest no significant differences in treatment outcomes depending on the delivery model. Our results demonstrate that the hybrid model can be applied in this patient group; however, the absence of a control group limits the ability to draw definitive conclusions.

4.1. Clinical Implications of the Inpatient Rehabilitation Protocol

In our group, all patients successfully completed the inpatient rehabilitation program. In 14 individuals (87%), a composite endpoint of mild clinical events was recorded after SNS. Our observations highlight the need for close postoperative monitoring, which may yield better treatment outcomes. This partially aligns with the findings of de Asmundis et al. (2024), who demonstrated that prophylactic use of aspirin and colchicine significantly reduced the incidence of symptomatic pericarditis after SNS [14]. In their study, pericarditis occurred in 18.1% of patients receiving prophylaxis, compared with 52.8% in the group without such treatment. In our series, despite the widespread use of colchicine, postpericardiotomy syndrome occurred relatively frequently. This suggests that preventive strategies still require further refinement. In contrast to the meta-analysis by Aerts et al. (2024) [25], who evaluated the short-term outcomes of isolated and hybrid thoracoscopic ablation in patients with atrial fibrillation, no major cardiovascular events or deaths were observed in our population of individuals with IST/POTS, indicating a favorable safety profile of this procedure. Furthermore, early cardiac rehabilitation appeared to enhance safety with continuous monitoring of clinical symptoms in the postoperative period. Meanwhile, the combination of gradual mobilization with physiological parameter assessment was associated with improved physical performance. These findings highlight the need to educate cardiologists and rehabilitation specialists about the SNS procedure, potential postoperative complications, and appropriate responses in emergencies. Implementing remote consultations involving a multidisciplinary HEART-TEAM may further improve care coordination. However, further comparative studies are needed to more precisely define the risks and benefits of this approach in different patient groups, which would allow the development of individualized treatment strategies. It may also be worth considering dedicated training for cardiologists and rehabilitation teams on the specifics of post-SNS care.

4.2. Insights from the Home-Based Telerehabilitation Protocol

In this study group, implementing telerehabilitation proved to be safe and well-accepted. Most participants (87%) completed the program, with the few dropouts being mainly due to medical or personal reasons. Although no formal statistical analysis was performed, preliminary observations—particularly during the third and sixth sessions—showed that individuals who ultimately achieved clinical improvement often rated their sessions as less tiring. This may suggest that an early, subjective perception of lower exertion could be an indicator of later clinical improvement. The flexibility of the model, allowing for individual adjustments to training intensity and type, likely contributed to its positive evaluation by participants [26]. Based on our experience, the hybrid rehabilitation model appears feasible to implement and may serve as an effective form of support for patients after SNS for IST or POTS.

4.3. Interpretation of the Clinical Assessment

In our group, the Malmö POTS scoring system turned out to be a useful tool for quantitatively assessing symptom severity. The mean score decreased from 65.3 before rehabilitation to 25.7 after its completion. This result suggests that the scale may be valuable in monitoring treatment effectiveness. It is also worth noting that the intervention contributed to a reduced mean heart rate, and in most patients, the therapeutic target of <90 beats/min was achieved. In our study, the resolution of the diagnostic criteria for IST/POTS was considered an early indicator of clinical improvement, although other studies (e.g., HEAL-IST) have applied different definitions of remission or patient improvement. It should also be noted that although 62% of participants achieved the target mean heart rate, the wide range of obtained values indicates significant individual variability in response to therapy. This underlines the need to tailor the rehabilitation program to each patient's profile and the importance of continuous heart rate monitoring with flexible adjustments to training intensity.

It should also be mentioned that not all patients may achieve complete remission without medication. As demonstrated in the HEAL-IST study, clinical improvement may occur later in the postprocedural period [9]. Symptom resolution can also be achieved by reintroducing pharmacological agents that were previously ineffective or poorly tolerated. Therefore, the absence of pharmacotherapy should not be the sole criterion for treatment success, and follow-up strategies should remain flexible, allowing for an individualized therapeutic approach.

4.4. Role of Psychological Support

A standardized psychological support program was introduced in cognitive behavioral methods with the assumption that in a post-surgical population, IST/POTS patients might show high levels of emotional reactivity and anxiety, particularly within early postoperative periods [27]. The organization of psychological care before and after the procedure most likely made it easier for patients to cooperate and be involved in rehabilitation. The findings emphasize the need for preoperative psychological support during recovery.

5. Limitations

Our study has several potential limitations. First, the sample size was relatively small and consisted of only women, which substantially limits both the statistical power and generalizability of the findings. However, it should be emphasized that the small number of participants reflects the early stage of SNS implementation in our region. For comparison, the only published experience from Central Europe to date includes only 20 patients (Stec et al., 2025) [28], which highlights the need for further regional research. We emphasize that this was a pilot study, initially designed to assess the feasibility, implementation, acceptance, and adherence of the HCR program. It is also worth noting that the sex distribution in our study reflects the epidemiological profile of IST/POTS, which predominantly affects younger women. Second, we acknowledge that the lack of a control group makes it difficult to precisely determine the extent to which the applied rehabilitation program contributed to the observed clinical improvement. Unfortunately, there is currently no standardized model of post-SNS care that could serve as a reference point. In most centers worldwide, post-procedure management solely relies on telemonitoring. In this context, our study offers a practical alternative care pathway and serves as a starting point for future multicenter studies with randomization or a control group. Third, in our group, there was only a single 6MWT, which does not allow objective evaluation of the physical performance in detection. However, it should be emphasized that the 6MWT was primarily used to determine the patient's baseline functional capacity and to individualize the training program in our study. Finally, it should be noted that patient-reported outcomes are inherently subjective, which in itself constitutes a limitation. Nevertheless, the Malmö POTS scoring system used in this study was selected for its standardization and validation, as well as its ability to better capture the spectrum of symptoms typical of IST/POTS. These data were supplemented with objective measurements, including ECG monitoring, and the active standing test performed two months after completing the HCR program.

6. Conclusions

Our hybrid HCR program—combining inpatient rehabilitation with home-based telerehabilitation—proved to be feasible, safe, and fully acceptable in patients with IST and POTS after SNS and was characterized by a high level of adherence. In our group, short-term follow-up revealed markedly reduced symptom severity and improved physical performance, which was also reflected in decreased Malmö POTS scores and better heart rate control. Although these results may suggest the potential effectiveness of combining personalized, structured rehabilitation with telemedicine tools in this specific patient group, the absence of a control group ultimately prevents us from drawing definitive conclusions. Further prospective, multicenter, controlled studies are needed to confirm our observations and determine their long-term effects [29].

Author Contributions: Conceptualization, M.K. (Marta Kornaszewska) and S.S.; Data curation, M.K. (Marta Kornaszewska), M.K. (Mariusz Kowalewski), N.O. and S.S.; Formal analysis, M.K. (Marta Kornaszewska), M.Z. and S.S.; Investigation, M.K. (Marta Kornaszewska), A.W.-B., A.R., B.S., M.K. (Mariusz Kowalewski), P.S., A.W. and S.S.; Methodology, M.K. (Marta Kornaszewska), A.W.-B., A.R., M.K. (Mariusz Kowalewski), P.S., M.Z. and S.S.; Project administration, M.K. (Marta Kornaszewska); Resources, M.K. (Marta Kornaszewska), A.W.-B., M.K. (Mariusz Kowalewski), P.S., N.O., A.W. and S.S.; Software, B.S. and M.P.; Supervision, E.P. and S.S.; Validation, M.K. (Marta Kornaszewska) and S.S.; Visualization, M.K. (Marta Kornaszewska), M.Z., M.P. and S.S.; Writing—original draft, M.K. (Marta Kornaszewska) and S.S.; Writing—review and editing, M.K. (Marta Kornaszewska), A.W.-B., A.R., E.P., B.S., M.K. (Mariusz Kowalewski), P.S., N.O., A.W., M.Z., M.P. and S.S. All authors have read and agreed to the published version of the manuscript.

Funding: This research received no external funding.

Institutional Review Board Statement: This study was approved by the Ethics Committee of the University of Rzeszow (decision number 5/4/2017-RARE-A-CAREgistry, 6 April 2017) and conducted in accordance with the Declaration of Helsinki.

Informed Consent Statement: Informed consent was obtained from all subjects involved in the study.

Data Availability Statement: Data are available from the corresponding author upon reasonable request. Due to privacy restrictions and the sensitive nature of patient data, the datasets generated and/or analyzed during the current study are not publicly available.

Acknowledgments: Logistic and IT support was kindly provided by The Institute for Cardiovascular Science CardioNeuroLab CardioMedicum, Cracow, Poland, and the DrEryk team.

Conflicts of Interest: Sebastian Stec is a cofounder and shareholder of Medicine S.A.; the author of six patents in cardiovascular medicine; no products have been used for this case. Piotr Suwalski serves as a consultant for AtriCure. No other conflicts of interest are relevant to the current study.

References

1. Mayuga, K.A.; Fedorowski, A.; Ricci, F.; Gopinathannair, R.; Dukes, J.W.; Gibbons, C.; Hanna, P.; Sorajja, D.; Chung, M.; Benditt, D.; et al. Sinus Tachycardia: A Multidisciplinary Expert Focused Review. *Circ. Arrhythm. Electrophysiol.* **2022**, *15*, e007960. [CrossRef]
2. Fedorowski, A.; Fanciulli, A.; Raj, S.R.; Sheldon, R.; Shibao, C.A.; Sutton, R. Cardiovascular autonomic dysfunction in post-COVID-19 syndrome: A major health-care burden. *Nat. Rev. Cardiol.* **2024**, *21*, 379–395. [CrossRef]
3. Fu, Q.; Levine, B.D. Exercise and non-pharmacological treatment of POTS. *Auton. Neurosci.* **2018**, *215*, 20–27. [CrossRef]
4. Abed, H.S.; Fulcher, J.R.; Kilborn, M.J.; Keech, A.C. Inappropriate sinus tachycardia: Focus on ivabradine. *Intern. Med. J.* **2016**, *46*, 875–883. [CrossRef]
5. Ahmed, A.; Pothineni, N.V.K.; Charate, R.; Garg, J.; Elbey, M.; de Asmundis, C.; LaMeir, M.; Romeya, A.; Shivamurthy, P.; Olshansky, B.; et al. Inappropriate Sinus Tachycardia: Etiology, Pathophysiology, and Management: JACC Review Topic of the Week. *J. Am. Coll. Cardiol.* **2022**, *79*, 2450–2462. [CrossRef]
6. Kanjwal, K.; Karabin, B.; Sheikh, M.; Elmer, L.; Kanjwal, Y.; Saeed, B.; Grubb, B.P. Pyridostigmine in the treatment of postural orthostatic tachycardia: A single-center experience. *Pacing Clin. Electrophysiol.* **2011**, *34*, 750–755. [CrossRef]
7. Lakkireddy, D.; Garg, J.; DeAsmundis, C.; LaMeier, M.; Romeya, A.; Vanmeetren, J.; Park, P.; Tummala, R.; Koerber, S.; Vasamreddy, C.; et al. Sinus Node Sparing Hybrid Thoracoscopic Ablation Outcomes in Patients with Inappropriate Sinus Tachycardia (SUSRUTA-IST) Registry. *Heart Rhythm* **2022**, *19*, 30–38. [CrossRef]

8. de Asmundis, C.; Chierchia, G.B.; Lakkireddy, D.; Romeya, A.; Okum, E.; Gandhi, G.; Sieira, J.; Vloka, M.; Jones, S.D.; Shah, H. et al. Sinus node sparing novel hybrid approach for treatment of inappropriate sinus tachycardia/postural sinus tachycardia Multicenter experience. *J. Interv. Card. Electrophysiol.* **2022**, *63*, 531–544. [CrossRef]
9. de Asmundis, C.; Pannone, L.; Lakkireddy, D.; Beaver, T.M.; Brodt, C.R.; Lee, R.J.; Frazier, K.; Chierchia, G.-B.; La Meir, M. Hybrid epicardial and endocardial sinus node-sparing ablation therapy for inappropriate sinus tachycardia: Rationale and design of the multicenter HEAL-IST IDE trial. *Heart Rhythm O2* **2023**, *4*, 275–282. [CrossRef]
10. Spahic, J.M.; Hamrefors, V.; Johansson, M.; Ricci, F.; Melander, O.; Sutton, R.; Fedorowski, A. Malmö POTS symptom score: Assessing symptom burden in postural orthostatic tachycardia syndrome. *J. Intern. Med.* **2023**, *293*, 91–99. [CrossRef] [PubMed]
11. Fedorowski, A. Postural orthostatic tachycardia syndrome: Clinical presentation, aetiology and management. *J. Intern. Med.* **2019**, *285*, 352–366. [CrossRef]
12. Page, R.L.; Joglar, J.A.; Caldwell, M.A.; Calkins, H.; Conti, J.B.; Deal, B.J.; Mark Estes, N.A., III; Field, M.E.; Goldberger, Z.D.; Hammill, S.C.; et al. 2015 ACC/AHA/HRS Guideline for the Management of Adult Patients With Supraventricular Tachycardia: Executive Summary: A Report of the American College of Cardiology/American Heart Association Task Force on Clinical Practice Guidelines and the Heart Rhythm Society. *Circulation* **2016**, *133*, e471–e505, Erratum in *Circulation* **2016**, *134*, e232–e233. [CrossRef] [PubMed]
13. Brugada, J.; Katritsis, D.G.; Arbelo, E.; Arribas, F.; Bax, J.J.; Blomström-Lundqvist, C.; Calkins, H.; Corrado, D.; Deftereos, S.G.; Diller, G.P.; et al. 2019 ESC Guidelines for the management of patients with supraventricular tachycardia The Task Force for the management of patients with supraventricular tachycardia of the European Society of Cardiology (ESC). *Eur. Heart J.* **2020**, *41*, 655–720, Erratum in *Eur. Heart J.* **2020**, *41*, 4258. [CrossRef]
14. de Asmundis, C.; Marcon, L.; Pannone, L.; Della Rocca, D.G.; Lakkireddy, D.; Beaver, T.M.; Brodt, C.R.; Monaco, C.; Sorgente, A.; Audiat, C.; et al. Pericarditis prophylactic therapy after sinus node-sparing hybrid ablation for inappropriate sinus tachycardia/postural orthostatic sinus tachycardia. *Heart Rhythm O2* **2024**, *5*, 137–144. [CrossRef] [PubMed]
15. Pelliccia, A.; Sharma, S.; Gati, S.; Bäck, M.; Börjesson, M.; Caselli, S.; Collet, J.P.; Corrado, D.; Drezner, J.A.; Halle, M.; et al. 2020 ESC Guidelines on sports cardiology and exercise in patients with cardiovascular disease. *Eur. Heart J.* **2021**, *42*, 17–96, Erratum in *Eur. Heart J.* **2021**, *42*, 548–549. [CrossRef] [PubMed]
16. Piepoli, M.F.; Conraads, V.; Corrà, U.; Dickstein, K.; Francis, D.P.; Jaarsma, T.; McMurray, J.; Pieske, B.; Piotrowicz, E.; Schmid, J.-P.; et al. Exercise training in heart failure: From theory to practice. A consensus document of the Heart Failure Association and the European Association for Cardiovascular Prevention and Rehabilitation. *Eur. J. Heart Fail.* **2011**, *13*, 347–357. [CrossRef] [PubMed]
17. Taylor, J.L.; Myers, J.; Bonikowske, A.R. Practical guidelines for exercise prescription in patients with chronic heart failure. *Heart Fail. Rev.* **2023**, *28*, 1285–1296. [CrossRef]
18. Piotrowicz, E.; Zieliński, T.; Bodalski, R.; Rywik, T.; Dobraszkiewicz-Wasilewska, B.; Sobieszczańska-Małek, M.; Stepnowska, M.; Przybylski, A.; Browarek, A.; Szumowski, Ł.; et al. Home-based telemonitored Nordic walking training is well accepted, safe, effective and has high adherence among heart failure patients, including those with cardiovascular implantable electronic devices: A randomised controlled study. *Eur. J. Prev. Cardiol.* **2015**, *22*, 1368–1377. [CrossRef]
19. Antoniou, V.; Davos, C.H.; Kapreli, E.; Batalik, L.; Panagiotakos, D.B.; Pepera, G. Effectiveness of Home-Based Cardiac Rehabilitation, Using Wearable Sensors, as a Multicomponent, Cutting-Edge Intervention: A Systematic Review and Meta-Analysis. *J. Clin. Med.* **2022**, *11*, 3772. [CrossRef]
20. Piotrowicz, E.; Mierzyńska, A.; Jaworska, I.; Opolski, G.; Banach, M.; Zaręba, W.; Kowalik, I.; Pencina, M.; Orzechowski, P.; Szalewska, D.; et al. Relationship between physical capacity and depression in heart failure patients undergoing hybrid comprehensive telerehabilitation vs. usual care: Subanalysis from the TELEREH-HF Randomized Clinical Trial. *Eur. J. Cardiovasc. Nurs.* **2022**, *21*, 568–577. [CrossRef]
21. Grubb, B.P.; Kanjwal, Y.; Kosinski, D.J. The postural tachycardia syndrome: A concise guide to diagnosis and management. *J. Cardiovasc. Electrophysiol.* **2006**, *17*, 108–112. [CrossRef]
22. Hou, C.R.; Olshansky, B.; Cortez, D.; Duval, S.; Benditt, D.G. Inappropriate sinus tachycardia: An examination of existing definitions. *Europace* **2022**, *24*, 1655–1664. [CrossRef]
23. Stec, S.; Suwalski, P.; De Asmundis, C.; La Meir, M.; Reichert, A.; Wilczek-Banc, A.; Szkaradek, B.; Kowalewski, M. EP-Heart Team approach with sinus node sparing ablation for complex inappropriate sinus tachycardia and postural orthostatic tachycardia syndrome: A first experience in Central Europe. *Kardiol. Pol.* **2025**, *83*, 342–344. [CrossRef]
24. Taylor, R.S.; Blakemore, A. Exercise-based cardiac rehabilitation: The importance of home-based approaches. *Eur. Heart J.* **2025**, *46*, 2202–2204. [CrossRef] [PubMed]
25. Aerts, L.; Kawczynski, M.J.; Bidar, E.; Luermans, J.G.L.; Chaldoupi, S.-M.; La Meir, M.; Kowalewski, M.; Maessen, J.G.; Heuts, S.; Maesen, B. Short- and long-term outcomes in isolated vs. hybrid thoracoscopic ablation in patients with atrial fibrillation: A systematic review and reconstructed individual patient data meta-analysis. *Europace* **2024**, *26*, euae232. [CrossRef] [PubMed]

26. Jafri, S.H.; Guglin, M.; Rao, R.; Ilonze, O.; Ballut, K.; Baloch, Z.Q.; Qintar, M.; Cohn, J.; Wilcox, M.; Freeman, A.M.; et al. Intensive Cardiac Rehabilitation Outcomes in Patients with Heart Failure. *J. Clin. Med.* **2023**, *12*, 6886. [CrossRef] [PubMed]
27. El-Rhermoul, F.-Z.; Fedorowski, A.; Eardley, P.; Taraborrelli, P.; Panagopoulos, D.; Sutton, R.; Lim, P.B.; Dani, M. Autoimmunity in Long Covid and POTS. *Oxf. Open Immunol.* **2023**, *4*, iqad002. [CrossRef]
28. Stec, S.; Suwalski, P.; de Asmundis, C.; LaMeir, M.; Kwaśniak, E.; Ogorzelec, N.; Reichert, A.; Wilczek-Banc, A.; Szkaradek, B.; Kowalewski, M. Hybrid sinus node sparing ablation for complex inappropriate sinus tachycardia and postural orthostatic tachycardia syndrome: Initial experience in Central Europe. *Pol. Arch. Intern. Med.* **2025**, *135*, 17014. [CrossRef]
29. Heindl, B.; Ramirez, L.; Joseph, L.; Clarkson, S.; Thomas, R.; Bittner, V. Hybrid cardiac rehabilitation—The state of the science and the way forward. *Prog. Cardiovasc. Dis.* **2022**, *70*, 175–182. [CrossRef]

Journal of
Clinical Medicine

MDPI

Article

Effectiveness and Safety of Hybrid Comprehensive Telerehabilitation in Women with Heart Failure—A Subanalysis of the TELEREH-HF Randomized Clinical Trial

Ewa Piotrowicz [1,*], Renata Główczyńska [2], Dominika Szalewska [3], Ilona Kowalik [4], Piotr Orzechowski [1], Sławomir Pluta [5], Zbigniew Kalarus [5], Anna Mierzyńska [4], Izabela Jaworska [5], Robert Irzmański [6] and Ryszard Piotrowicz [4]

1 Telecardiology Center, National Institute of Cardiology, 04-628 Warsaw, Poland; porzechowski@ikard.pl
2 1st Chair and Department of Cardiology, Medical University of Warsaw, 02-097 Warsaw, Poland
3 Clinic of Rehabilitation Medicine, Faculty of Health Sciences, Medical University of Gdańsk, 80-210 Gdańsk, Poland
4 National Institute of Cardiology, 04-628 Warsaw, Poland; rpiotrowicz@ikard.pl (R.P.)
5 Department of Cardiology, Congenital Heart Diseases and Electrotherapy, Silesian Center for Heart Diseases, Silesian Medical University, 41-800 Zabrze, Poland; i.jaworska@sccs.pl (I.J.)
6 Department of Internal Medicine and Cardiac Rehabilitation, Medical University of Łódź, 90-647 Łódź, Poland
* Correspondence: epiotrowicz@ikard.pl

Abstract

Background/Objectives: Despite the known benefits of cardiac rehabilitation, it remains underutilized among women. In particular, little is known about the effectiveness of hybrid comprehensive telerehabilitation (HCTR) in women with heart failure (HF). The purpose of this study was to assess effectiveness and safety of HCTR in women with HF. **Methods**: This analysis formed part of the TELEREH-HF multicenter, randomized trial that enrolled 850 HF patients (NYHA I-III, LVEF $\leq$ 40%). Patients were randomized 1:1 to HCTR plus usual care (UC) or UC alone. Patients underwent either HCTR (1 week in hospital and 8 weeks at home, five times weekly) or UC with observation. The effectiveness of HCTR was assessed by changes in peak oxygen consumption (VO_2peak), workload duration (t) in cardiopulmonary exercise test and quality of life (QoL) based on Medical Outcome Survey Short Form 36 Questionnaire (SF-36). Measurements were taken before and after intervention/observation. **Results**: Women constituted 11.5% of the TELEREH-HF study population. Forty women in the HCTR group and 44 women in the UC group completed program and observation, respectively. HCTR resulted in a significant improvement in VO_2peak (13.4 $\pm$ 4.3 vs. 14.3 $\pm$ 4.6; 95%CI 0.91 [0.05; 1.77], p = 0.038), workload duration (301 $\pm$ 162.3 vs. 334 $\pm$ 156.6; 95%CI 33 [5; 60], p = 0.022) and SF-36 overall score (85.9 $\pm$ 13.6 vs. 89.9 $\pm$ 13.5; 95%CI 4.0 [0.6; 7.4], p = 0.024). These favorable results were not observed in the UC group VO_2peak (14.2 $\pm$ 4.8 vs. 14.2 $\pm$ 4.8; 95%CI 0.02 [−1.20; 1.24], p = 0.971) and SF-36 overall score (89.1 $\pm$ 17.4 vs. 89.5 $\pm$ 15.8; 95%CI 4.0 [−2.1; 2.8], p = 0.796), except for an increase workload duration (268 $\pm$ 138.4 vs. 300 $\pm$ 130.1; 95%CI 32 [2; 62], p = 0.036). The HCTR group showed a significantly greater improvement in the physical component of QoL than the UC group. In neither group were there deaths nor major adverse events related to exercise training. **Conclusions**: Among women with heart failure, hybrid comprehensive telerehabilitation appears safe and leads to statistically significant although moderate improvements in physical capacity and quality of life. However, due to the small sample size, further studies in larger female populations are needed to confirm these findings.

 https://doi.org/10.3390/jcm15020694

Keywords: women; hybrid telerehabilitation; heart failure with reduced ejection fraction

1. Introduction

Heart failure (HF) remains a major public health concern, with significant clinical, psychological, and economic consequences. Women with HF often present with more severe symptoms, lower exercise tolerance, and reduced health-related quality of life (QoL) compared to men, yet they are markedly underrepresented in cardiac rehabilitation programmes [1,2]. Despite strong recommendations in clinical guidelines, cardiac rehabilitation remains underutilised—particularly among female patients—due to factors such as caregiving responsibilities, limited referrals, and restricted access to facility-based services [3,4].

Comprehensive cardiac rehabilitation is a cornerstone of secondary prevention in cardiovascular disease and plays a critical role in improving outcomes in HF [3–7]. Alternative models such as hybrid comprehensive telerehabilitation (HCTR) have been developed to address the barriers limiting participation, especially among women. HCTR is an intervention that combines elements of conventional, in-center cardiac rehabilitation with remote, technology-assisted components. Its concept is based on the integration of two forms of rehabilitation: initially supervised in-center sessions, followed by remotely monitored home-based training sessions during which ECG, target training heart rate, blood pressure, and body mass are monitored. Core components typically include individualized exercise training, educational modules on lifestyle and disease management, regular monitoring of physiological parameters, and structured follow-up care via telecommunication. HCTR differs from conventional cardiac rehabilitation by offering greater flexibility and accessibility through remote components while retaining the benefits of direct professional supervision. Compared with fully remote programs, HCTR retains an in-person component, allowing for hands-on assessment and individualized rehabilitation planning. This model has the potential to increase accessibility, adherence, and long-term engagement in cardiac rehabilitation, particularly among underserved populations [5].

The TELEREH-HF randomised controlled trial demonstrated that HCTR improves functional capacity and QoL in patients with HF with reduced ejection fraction (HFrEF), and that it is safe and feasible for broader clinical implementation [6,8,9]. However, the specific effects of this intervention in women remain unclear due to their low representation in previous studies. Sex-specific evaluations are essential to ensure equitable, evidence-based care. In particular, little is known about the effectiveness of HCTR in women with HF. Therefore, the purpose of this subanalysis of the TELEREH-HF trial was to assess effectiveness and safety of HCTR in women with HF. The primary objective of this subanalysis was to evaluate the impact of HCTR on functional capacity, as measured by peak VO_2 and exercise duration, and on quality of life, assessed using the SF-36 questionnaire. The secondary objective was to evaluate the safety of the intervention.

2. Materials and Methods

The present analysis formed part of TELEREH-HF randomized, multi-center (five centers in Poland), prospective, open-label, parallel-group, controlled study (Clinical Trials.gov NCT 02523560), which enrolled 850 HF patients (New York Heart Association [NYHA] I-III, left ventricular ejection fraction [LVEF] $\leq$ 40%) who had been hospitalized for worsening HF within six months prior to randomization. Patients were randomized 1:1 to receive HCTR plus usual care (UC) or UC alone. The first patient was recruited on 31 August 2015.

https://doi.org/10.3390/jcm15020694

Patients underwent either the HCTR program—which consisted of one week in hospital, followed by eight weeks of home-based training performed five times weekly—or UC with observation. The HCTR intervention was comprehensive and included telecare, tailored home-based telerehabilitation, and remote monitoring of cardiovascular implantable electronic devices. The rehabilitation regimen comprised personalized endurance aerobic training based on Nordic walking, respiratory muscle training, and light resistance and strength exercises. Dietary consultation and interactive nutrition education were conducted in a group format on-site at the center. Additionally, patients were provided with access to the project's website, where information regarding diet was available. Patients randomized to the UC group were observed and received UC appropriate to their clinical status at their respective centers.

The design, the inclusion and exclusion criteria, the detailed description of the medical team composition, telemonitoring equipment, intervention protocols and primary results of the TELEREH-HF study have been published elsewhere [8–12].

The study adhered to good clinical practice guidelines and was conducted in accordance with the Declaration of Helsinki and applicable Polish regulations. The trial protocol was approved by the local ethics committee (IK-NP-0021-85/1402/13) and all patients provided written informed consent [8,9].

All patients underwent clinical examination, laboratory testing, echocardiography, cardiopulmonary exercise testing (CPET), and psychological assessment both at baseline and after completing the nine-week program.

2.1. Cardiopulmonary Exercise Test

The symptom-limited CPET on a treadmill according to a ramp protocol and the ESC guidelines was performed using a Schiller MTM-1500 med; Schiller, Baar, Switzerland [13,14]. Oxygen consumption (VO_2) was measured continuously using breath-by-breath analysis. The peak VO_2 value was presented per kilogram of body mass per minute (mL/kg/min). Maximal exercise was defined as the respiratory exchange ratio (RER) ≥ 1.

2.2. Health-Related Quality of Life Assessment

The Medical Outcome Survey Short Form 36 Questionnaire (SF-36) was used to assess QoL. The SF-36 consists of two major domains (physical and mental QoL) and various subscales [15]. Higher scores indicate a better QoL. We chose the SF-36 because this questionnaire provides detailed information on both physical and mental health domains, which was particularly relevant for our study assessing the broader impact of HCTR.

The effectiveness of HCTR was assessed by changes delta (Δ) in peak VO_2, workload duration (t) in CPET and QoL based on SF-36. Measurements were made before and after intervention/observation.

2.3. Statistical Analyses

Numerical variables are presented as means and SD or median and interquartile ranges (IQR), as appropriate. The distribution of data was examined by the Shapiro–Wilks test. Depending on the distribution comparisons between groups were made using Student's *t*-test or the Mann–Whitney test. For comparisons within groups, appropriate paired tests were used: paired Student's *t*-test or the Wilcoxon signed-rank test. Categorical variables are shown as counts and percentages. The χ^2-test or Fisher's exact test was performed to verify equality of proportions. 95% confidence intervals (Cis) were calculated for changes in VO_2, workload duration, and quality of life. Cohen's d was used as the measure of effect size, with 0.2 considered a weak effect, 0.5 a moderate effect, and 0.8 a strong effect. Due to the small size of the subgroups (this analysis represents a sub-study), complex analysis designs were not used, and no correction for multiple comparisons was made. All tests

 https://doi.org/10.3390/jcm15020694

were two-sided, and a p-value < 0.05 was considered statistically significant. All analyses were conducted using SAS software version 9.4.

3. Results

Of the 850 patients randomized to TELEREH-HF trial, 425 were assigned to the HCTR group and 425 to the UC group. Women constituted 11.5% of study population (48 in the HCTR group and 49 in the UC group). There were 2 women among the 27 patients who did not undergo telerehabilitation. One woman was unable to participate due to technical difficulties operating the telerehabilitation equipment, and the other due to new-onset comorbidities.

Among the 46 women who started telerehabilitation, five discontinued HCTR due to returning to work, and one died following postoperative complications (unrelated to the intervention). This subanalysis ultimately included 40 women in the HCTR group who completed the 9-week hybrid telerehabilitation program and 44 women in the UC group who completed the observation period Figure 1. Adherence to the 9-week HCTR program was high—approximately 89%.

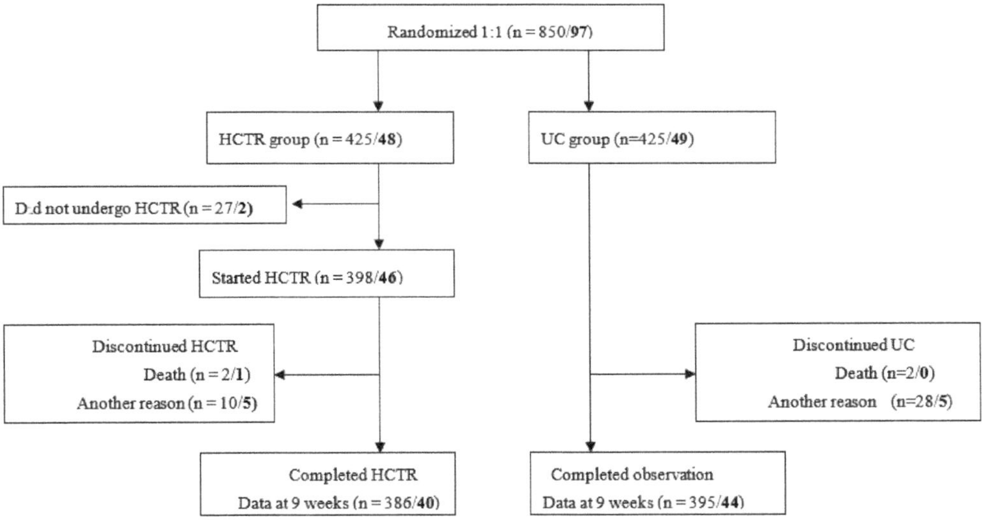

Figure 1. Flow of the entire patient population/women through the TELERH-HF study. HCTR—hybrid comprehensive telerehabilitation, UC—usual care.

The baseline characteristics of women in both groups (HCTR and UC) enrolled in the TELEREH-HF trial are presented in Table 1. Neither sodium–glucose cotransporter-2 (SGLT2) inhibitors nor glucagon-like peptide-1 (GLP-1) receptor agonists were used in the study population. The randomization and intervention/observation period took place before these drug classes became part of guideline-recommended therapy for HF; therefore, none of the participants received these medications. No significant differences were observed between groups at baseline in demographic data, clinical parameters, or treatment. The mean age of women was relatively low in both groups (58.8 years in HCTR; 63.0 years in UC; $p = 0.089$) and LVEF was 31.9% and 33.8% in the HCTR and UC groups, respectively ($p = 0.153$). Ischemic etiology of HF was diagnosed with comparable frequency: 40% in the HCTR group vs. 47.7% in the UC group ($p = 0.476$).

https://doi.org/10.3390/jcm15020694

Table 1. Baseline characteristics.

	HCTR Group (n = 40)	UC Group (n = 44)	p
Age (years). mean ± SD	58.8 ± 13.3	63.0 ± 8.3	0.089
Left Ventricular Ejection Fraction (%). mean ± SD	31.9 ± 6.6	33.8 ± 5.5	0.153
Body Mass Index (kg/m^2)	27.8 ± 5.9	28.6 ± 5.4	0.523
Body Mass Index (kg/m^2) ≤ 25.0	14 (35.0)	13 (29.5)	0.855
Body Mass Index (kg/m^2) > 25.0 < 30.0	14 (35.0)	16 (36.4)	
Body Mass Index (kg/m^2) ≥ 30.0	12 (30.0)	15 (34.1)	
Atrial fibrillation or atrial flutter. n (%)	5 (12.5%)	5 (11.4)	1.00
Etiology of heart failure. n (%)			
Ischaemic	16 (40.0)	21 (47.7)	0.476
Non-ischaemic	24 (60.0)	23 (52.3)	
Coronary artery disease	16 (40.0)	20 (45.4)	0.614
Myocardial infarction	15 (37.5)	19 (43.2)	0.596
Angioplasty	13 (32.5)	15 (34.1)	0.877
Coronary artery bypass grafting	3 (7.5)	3 (6.8)	1.00
Hypertension	22 (55.0)	25 (56.8)	0.867
Diabetes	9 (22.5)	12 (27.3)	0.614
Stroke	2 (5.0)	3 (6.8)	1.00
Chronic kidney disease	10 (25.0)	8 (18.2)	0.447
Hyperlipidemia	18 (45.0)	18 (40.9)	0.705
NYHA I. n (%)	2 (5.0)	2 (4.6)	0.845
NYHA II. n (%)	31 (77.5)	32 (72.7)	
NYHA III. n (%)	7 (17.5)	10 (22.7)	
Beta-blocker	38 (95.0)	42 (95.3)	1.00
ACEI/ARB	36 (90.0)	38 (86.4)	0.741
Digoxin	3 (7.5)	7 (15.9)	0.319
Loop diuretics	32 (80.0)	31 (70.4)	0.313
Spironolactone/eplerenone	33 (82.5)	31 (70.4)	0.195
Aspirin/clopidogrel	18 (45.0)	24 (54.5)	0.382
Anticoagulants	10 (25.0)	10 (22.7)	0.807
Statins	29 (72.5)	30 (68.2)	0.666
CIEDs	29 (72.5)	28 (63.6)	0.385
Implantable cardioverter–defibrillator	15 (51.7)	14 (50.0)	1.00
CRT-P	1 (3.4)	0 (0)	
CRT-D	12 (41.4)	13 (46.3)	
PM	1 (3.5)	1 (3.6)	

Abbreviations: NYHA—New York Heart Association class; ACEI—angiotensin-converting enzyme inhibitors; ARB—angiotensin receptor blockers; CIEDs—cardiovascular implantable electronic devices; CRT-P—cardiac resynchronization therapy; CRT-D—cardiac resynchronization therapy and cardioverter–defibrillator; PM—pacemaker.

Cardiopulmonary exercise test results and QoL scores at baseline and after the 9-week intervention/observation period are presented in Tables 2 and 3. At baseline the study groups did not differ significantly in workload duration and peak VO_2. In both groups workload duration improved significantly compared to baseline (p = 0.022 in HCTR and

https://doi.org/10.3390/jcm15020694

$p = 0.036$ in UC, respectively). HCTR also resulted in a significant improvement in peak VO_2 ($p = 0.038$), whereas no significant change in this parameter was observed in the UC group; so that in the HCTR group the increase in peak VO_2 after 9 weeks occurred in 29 patients (72.5%), while in the UC group only in 19 patients (46.3%), $p = 0.017$.

Table 2. Results—effectiveness of hybrid comprehensive telerehabilitation in women with heart failure.

Parameters	Hybrid Comprehensive Telerehabilitation (HCTR) Group				Usual Care (UC) Group			
	Baseline	9th Week	Δ [95% CI]	p	Baseline	9th Week	Δ [95% CI]	p
Workload duration (s)	301 ± 162.3	334 ± 156.6	33 [5; 60]	0.022	268 ± 138.4	300 ± 130.1	32 [2; 62]	0.036
peakVO$_2$ (mL/kg/min)	13.4 ± 4.7	14.3 ± 4.6	0.91 [0.05; 1.77]	0.038	14.2 ± 4.8	14.2 ± 4.8	0.02 [−1.20; 1.24]	0.971
SF36 Physical Component Score	39.8 ± 6.5	41.8 ± 6.7	2.0 [0.05; 3.9]	0.044	41.1 ± 8.7	40.4 ± 7.1	−0.7 [−2.1; 0.5]	0.239
SF36 Mental Component Score	46.1 ± 11.1	48.1± 10.1	2.0 [−0.5; 4.6]	0.118	48.0 ± 12.7	49.1 ± 11.5	1.1 [−1.2; 3.4]	0.338
SF 36—overall score	85.9 ± 13.6	89.9 ± 13.5	4.0 [0.6; 7.4]	0.024	89.1 ± 17.4	89.5 ± 15.8	0.4 [−2.1; 2.8]	0.796

SF-36—The Medical Outcome Survey Short Form 36 Questionnaire.

Table 3. Results—Cohen's d; effectiveness of hybrid comprehensive telerehabilitation in women with heart failure.

	Cohen's d	
Parameters	Hybrid Comprehensive Telerehabilitation (HCTR) Group	Usual Care (UC) Group
Workload duration (s)	0.38	0.33
peakVO$_2$ (mL/kg/min)	0.34	0.01
SF36 Physical Component Score	0.33	0.16
SF36 Mental Component Score	0.25	0.15
SF 36—overall score	0.37	0.05

SF-36—The Medical Outcome Survey Short Form 36 Questionnaire.

Following the intervention, the HCTR group showed a significant improvement in overall QoL compared to baseline (Δ = 4.0 [0.6; 7.4]; $p = 0.024$) and in the physical domain of QoL (Δ = 2.0 [0.05; 3.9]; $p = 0.044$). No significant changes were observed in the mental domain of QoL in the HCTR group. However, no statistically significant differences were found in overall QoL or its domains in the UC group after the observation period.

In the baseline assessment, the HCTR group included 35% of patients who were overweight and 30% who were obese; in the UC group, these proportions were 36.4% and 34.1%, respectively (Table 1). Among patients with overweight or obesity, body mass did not change significantly after the intervention/observation period in either group. In the HCTR group, median (Q1–Q3) body mass was 73 (64–84) kg at baseline and 74 (64–84) kg after 9 weeks ($p = 0.864$). In the UC group, the corresponding values were 74 (65–85) kg at baseline and 75 (64.5–85.5) kg after 9 weeks ($p = 0.811$).

No deaths or major adverse events related to exercise training occurred in either group.

4. Discussion

Cardiac rehabilitation is a well-established intervention proven to reduce recurrent cardiac events, enhance functional capacity, and improve QoL. In our study, we observed a significantly greater improvement in the physical component of QoL in the HCTR group compared with UC. The HCTR group achieved a significant increase in peak VO_2, demonstrating a clear enhancement in exercise capacity among women. Moreover, a substantially

https://doi.org/10.3390/jcm15020694

higher proportion of women in the HCTR group improved their peak VO_2 compared with those receiving UC, highlighting the superior functional benefits of the hybrid telerehabilitation approach. We found significant improvements in overall QoL and its physical domain in the HCTR group, whereas no such improvements were observed in the UC group; QoL in the mental domain remained unchanged in both groups. Importantly, in our study, the hybrid telerehabilitation program demonstrated an excellent safety profile, with no deaths or major exercise-related adverse events.

Although historically underrecognized, HF in women presents distinct epidemiological, pathophysiological, and clinical features compared to men. Women with HF often exhibit different symptoms, respond differently to treatments, and face unique psychosocial and healthcare access challenges. Understanding these differences is essential for developing effective, gender-sensitive diagnostic and therapeutic strategies.

Women develop HF later in life than men and more frequently exhibit non-ischemic etiologies such as hypertensive heart disease, valvular dysfunction, and HF with preserved ejection fraction (HFpEF). These phenotypes are often characterized by distinct symptom profiles, including greater dyspnea, fatigue, and exercise intolerance, which can complicate diagnosis and management.

Women with HF often report lower QoL and higher levels of depression and anxiety than their male counterparts. These psychosocial challenges can negatively impact self-care behaviors and adherence to treatment. Social support networks, counseling, and mental health care are therefore essential components of comprehensive HF management in women.

Given these differences, several mechanisms may underlie sex-specific responses to telerehabilitation. Biologically, HF phenotypes predominant in women—such as HFpEF and microvascular dysfunction—are marked by exercise intolerance and impaired peripheral oxygen extraction, which may respond particularly well to the progressive aerobic conditioning central to telerehabilitation. Sex-related differences in autonomic regulation, resting heart rate, heart rate variability, and thoracic anatomy may also influence how physiological signals are captured and interpreted by remote monitoring systems, potentially affecting the personalization of exercise loads. Psychosocial factors further shape women's engagement: higher levels of fatigue, anxiety, and depressive symptoms can hinder participation in traditional center-based programs, whereas the privacy and flexibility of home-based training may enhance emotional safety and comfort. In addition, caregiving duties and time constraints—a well-recognized burden for many women—are alleviated by the reduced travel and scheduling demands of telerehabilitation. Adherence-related mechanisms are also relevant. Though older women may initially express lower confidence with digital tools, structured education, intuitive interfaces, and regular feedback have been shown to improve digital competence and sustain engagement. Women often value frequent reassurance and personalized communication, and telehealth platforms that provide continuous feedback and support may strengthen motivation and adherence.

Extensive research consistently shows that cardiac rehabilitation reduces mortality, improves physical fitness, and enhances psychological well-being in both sexes [16]. For women specifically, it offers an opportunity to address modifiable risk factors such as hypertension, hyperlipidemia, diabetes, obesity, and depression—which are highly prevalent in female cardiovascular populations. Additionally, women more commonly present with non-obstructive coronary artery disease, microvascular dysfunction, and atypical symptoms, which may complicate diagnosis and management [17]. Cardiac rehabilitation provides a personalized and holistic framework well suited to addressing these gender-specific clinical nuances.

https://doi.org/10.3390/jcm15020694

Although cardiac rehabilitation is highly effective, women consistently participate less often than men. Referral biases, competing caregiving responsibilities, socioeconomic constraints, and psychological barriers, such as lower self-efficacy and fear of exercise contribute to this gap. Despite its benefits, traditional center-based cardiac rehabilitation faces notable challenges, including limited accessibility, low participation rates, and logistical difficulties-issues that disproportionately affect women. In our TELEREH-HF study, women represented only 11.5% of the population, with similar proportions in both the HCTR and UC groups, reflecting the well-documented underrepresentation of women in rehabilitation programs. Underrepresentation limits evidence-based, gender-informed decision-making and may contribute to poorer outcomes after cardiovascular events.

Several factors contribute to this disparity. Physicians may be less likely to refer women, particularly younger women or those presenting with atypical symptoms, to rehabilitation programs [4]. Sociocultural responsibilities, including caregiving and household duties, often restrict women's ability to attend scheduled sessions [18]. Additionally, higher rates of depression and anxiety, lower self-efficacy, and feelings of vulnerability can hinder women's participation and adherence [19]. Although cardiovascular disease remains the leading cause of death among women worldwide, they continue to be underreferred to and underrepresented in cardiac rehabilitation, frequently experiencing poorer post-event outcomes than men.

Cardiac rehabilitation, including structured exercise training, education, and counseling is a proven strategy for reducing mortality and improving QoL [20]. To maximize benefit for women, however, programs must address gender-specific physiological and psychosocial barriers. Understanding and reducing these obstacles is essential for improving rehabilitation engagement and outcomes among women.

Telerehabilitation, the remote delivery of cardiac rehabilitation through digital and telecommunication technologies, presents a promising and increasingly validated alternative. Remote monitoring and hybrid cardiac telerehabilitation offer promising strategies to reduce disparities, yet sex-specific performance data remain scarce. Physiological parameters commonly used in remote monitoring, such as heart rate variability, thoracic impedance, arrhythmia burden, and physical activity levels may differ between men and women. These variations could influence the accuracy and predictive value of telerehabilitation algorithms, which were predominantly validated in male populations [21].

Multiple studies have shown telerehabilitation to be comparable in effectiveness to traditional, center-based rehabilitation. A meta-analysis by Thomas et al. [22] demonstrated that digital home-based programs result in similar improvements in peak oxygen uptake, exercise capacity, and health-related QoL. In the TELEREH-HF study, we further confirmed that telerehabilitation can enhance physical capacity in women with HF, evidenced by increased peak VO_2 and prolonged workload duration.

Recent evidence also supports the broader effectiveness of telerehabilitation. A review by Jin et al. [23] reported that programs incorporating structured exercise, education, and behavioral counseling significantly improve physical activity levels and patient adherence compared to standard care. These findings reinforce the feasibility and clinical value of telerehabilitation across diverse patient groups.

Beyond clinical efficacy, telerehabilitation offers several practical advantages. It addresses geographic and transportation barriers, making it particularly suitable for individuals living in rural or underserved regions [24]. It also reduces travel-related burden, lowers facility and system costs, and has the potential to decrease hospital readmissions.

Flexible scheduling, reduced travel burden, and the ability to exercise in a home environment may improve participation and adherence. Findings from the TELEREH-HF study support these advantages: women in the HCTR group demonstrated significant

https://doi.org/10.3390/jcm15020694

improvement in exercise capacity, including increased peak VO_2 and prolonged workload duration. A greater proportion of women improved peak VO_2 compared with usual care, underscoring the superior functional benefit of HCTR. QoL also improved significantly, particularly in the physical domain, whereas no meaningful changes were observed among women receiving usual care.

Given the strong potential of telerehabilitation to reduce access barriers and enhance engagement, future research must incorporate balanced male–female representation and report sex-disaggregated outcomes. Such efforts are essential for ensuring that digital innovations in HF management benefit women equitably and improve long-term clinical trajectories.

Limitation. This study has several limitations that should be acknowledged. First, the sample size of female participants was relatively small, reflecting the overall underrepresentation of women in the TELEREH-HF trial. As a result, the statistical power to detect differences between groups may be limited, and findings should be interpreted with caution. Second, the study population consisted solely of patients from centers in Poland, which may limit the generalizability of the results to more diverse populations or healthcare settings. Third, psychological and social factors could influence participation and outcomes—such as motivation, support systems, or socioeconomic status—were not extensively assessed. Finally, the follow-up period was limited to nine weeks; therefore, the long-term effects of HCTR on clinical outcomes and QoL in women with HF remain unknown and warrant further investigation. Furthermore, this subanalysis was conducted post hoc, which limits the interpretability of the results. The study was open-label by design; therefore, a limitation is the lack of blinding of outcome assessors, which would have reduced potential bias.

5. Conclusions

Among women with heart failure, hybrid comprehensive telerehabilitation appears safe and leads to statistically significant although moderate improvements in physical capacity and quality of life. However, due to the small sample size, further studies in larger female populations are needed to confirm these findings.

Author Contributions: Conceptualization, E.P. and R.P.; methodology, E.P. and R.P.; software, I.K.; validation, E.P., I.K. and R.P.; formal analysis, I.K.; investigation, E.P., R.G., D.S., P.O., S.P., A.M., I.J. and R.I.; resources, E.P.; data curation, I.K.; writing—original draft preparation, E.P., R.G. and D.S.; writing—review and editing, E.P., R.G., D.S., P.O., S.P., Z.K., A.M., I.J., R.I. and R.P.; visualization, E.P.; supervision, R.P.; project administration, E.P.; funding acquisition, E.P. All authors have read and agreed to the published version of the manuscript.

Funding: The study was financed by the National Centre for Research and Development, Warsaw, Poland (grant number STRATEGMED1/233547/13/NCBR/2015). The authors are solely responsible for the design and implementation of this study, all analyses, the drafting and editing of the paper, and its final content.

Institutional Review Board Statement: The study was conducted in accordance with the Declaration of Helsinki and approved by the Ethics Committee of Institute of Cardiology in Warsaw (protocol code IK-NP-0021-85/1402/13, date: 5 November 2013).

Informed Consent Statement: Informed consent was obtained from all subjects involved in the study.

Data Availability Statement: The data used to support the findings of this study are included within the article.

Conflicts of Interest: The authors declare no conflict of interest.

https://doi.org/10.3390/jcm15020694

Abbreviations

The following abbreviations are used in this manuscript:

HF	Heart Failure
QoL	Quality of life
HCTR	Hybrid Comprehensive TeleRehabilitation
LVEF	Left Ventricular Ejection Fraction
UC	Usual Care
CPET	CardioPulmonary Exercise Test
NYHA	New York Heart Association
SF-36	Medical Outcome Survey Short Form 36 Questionnaire

References

1. Dunlay, S.M.; Roger, V.L. Gender differences in the pathophysiology, clinical presentation, and outcomes of heart failure. *Curr. Heart Fail. Rep.* **2012**, *9*, 242–249. [CrossRef]
2. O'Connor, C.M.; Whellan, D.J.; Lee, K.L.; Keteyian, S.J.; Cooper, L.S.; Ellis, S.J.; Leifer, E.S.; Kraus, W.E.; Kitzman, D.W.; Blumenthal, J.A.; et al. Efficacy and safety of exercise training in patients with chronic heart failure: HF-ACTION randomized controlled trial. *J. Am. Med. Assoc.* **2009**, *301*, 1439–1450. [CrossRef]
3. McDonagh, T.A.; Metra, M.; Adamo, M.; Gardner, R.S.; Baumbach, A.; Böhm, M.; Burri, H.; Butler, J.; Čelutkienė, J.; Chioncel, O.; et al. 2021 ESC Guidelines for the diagnosis and treatment of acute and chronic heart failure. *Eur. Heart J.* **2021**, *42*, 3599–3726. [CrossRef]
4. Sanderson, B.K.; Bittner, V. Women in cardiac rehabilitation: Outcomes and identifying risk for dropout. *Am. Heart J.* **2005**, *150*, 1052–1058. [CrossRef] [PubMed]
5. Piotrowicz, E. How to do: Telerehabilitation in heart failure patients. *Cardiol. J.* **2012**, *19*, 243–248. [CrossRef] [PubMed]
6. Szalewska, D.; Główczyńska, R.; Piotrowicz, R.; Kowalik, I.; Pencina, M.J.; Opolski, G.; Zaręba, W.; Banach, M.; Orzechowski, P.; Pluta, S.; et al. An aetiology-based subanalysis of the Telerehabilitation in Heart Failure Patients (TELEREH-HF) trial. *ESC Heart Fail.* **2021**, *8*, 1263–1273. [CrossRef] [PubMed]
7. Piepoli, M.F.; Conraads, V.; Corra, U.; Dickstein, K.; Francis, D.P.; Jaarsma, T.; McMurray, J.; Pieske, B.; Piotrowicz, E.; Schmid, J.P.; et al. Exercise training in heart failure: From theory to practice. A consensus document of the Heart Failure Association and the European Association for Cardiovascular Prevention and Rehabilitation. *Eur. J. Heart Fail.* **2011**, *13*, 347–357. [CrossRef]
8. Piotrowicz, E.; Piotrowicz, R.; Opolski, G.; Pencina, M.; Banach, M.; Zaręba, W. Hybrid comprehensive telerehabilitation in heart failure patients (TELEREH-HF): A randomized, multicenter, prospective, open-label, parallel group controlled trial-Study design and description of the intervention. *Am. Heart J.* **2019**, *217*, 148–158. [CrossRef] [PubMed]
9. Piotrowicz, E.; Pencina, M.J.; Opolski, G.; Zaręba, W.; Banach, M.; Kowalik, I.; Orzechowski, P.; Szalewska, D.; Pluta, S.; Główczyńska, R.; et al. Effects of a 9-Week Hybrid Comprehensive Telerehabilitation Program on Long-term Outcomes in Patients With Heart Failure: The Telerehabilitation in Heart Failure Patients (TELEREH-HF) Randomized Clinical Trial. *J. Am. Med. Assoc. Cardiol.* **2020**, *5*, 300–308. [CrossRef] [PubMed]
10. Piotrowicz, E.; Mierzyńska, A.; Banach, M.; Jaworska, I.; Pencina, M.; Kowalik, I.; Pluta, S.; Szalewska, D.; Opolski, G.; Zaręba, W.; et al. Quality of life in heart failure patients undergoing hybrid comprehensive telerehabilitation versus usual care—Results of the Telerehabilitation in Heart Failure Patients (TELEREH-HF) Randomized Clinical Trial. *Arch. Med. Sci.* **2021**, *17*, 1599–1612. [CrossRef] [PubMed]
11. Główczyńska, R.; Piotrowicz, E.; Szalewska, D.; Piotrowicz, R.; Kowalik, I.; Pencina, M.J.; Zaręba, W.; Banach, M.; Orzechowski, P.; Pluta, S.; et al. Effects of hybrid comprehensive telerehabilitation on cardiopulmonary capacity in heart failure patients depending on diabetes mellitus: Subanalysis of the TELEREH-HF randomized clinical trial. *Cardiovasc. Diabetol.* **2021**, *20*, 106. [CrossRef]
12. Niewada, M.; Tabor, B.; Piotrowicz, E.; Piotrowicz, R.; Opolski, G.; Banach, M.; Jakubczyk, M. Cost-effectiveness of telerehabilitation in patients with heart failure in Poland: An analysis based on the results of Telerehabilitation in the Heart Failure Patients (TELEREH-HF) randomized clinical trial. *Kardiol. Pol.* **2021**, *79*, 510–516. [CrossRef] [PubMed]
13. Balady, G.J. Medical Evaluation and Exercise Testing. In *Guidelines for Cardiac Rehabilitation and Secondary Prevention Programs*, 4th ed.; Williams, M.A., Ed.; Human Kinetics: Champaign, IL, USA, 2004; Volume 79.
14. Piepoli, M.F.; Corrà, U.; Agostoni, P.G.; Belardinelli, R.; Cohen-Solal, A.; Hambrecht, R.; Vanhees, L.; Task Force of the Italian Working Group on Cardiac Rehabilitation and Prevention (Gruppo Italiano di Cardiologia Riabilitativa e Prevenzione, GICR); Working Group on Cardiac Rehabilitation and Exercise Physiology of the European Society of Cardiology. Statement on cardiopulmonary exercise testing in chronic heart failure due to left ventricular dysfunction: Recommendations for performance and interpretation Part II: How to perform cardiopulmonary exercise testing in chronic heart failure. *Eur. J. Cardiovasc. Prev. Rehabil.* **2006**, *13*, 300–311. [CrossRef] [PubMed]

https://doi.org/10.3390/jcm15020694

15. Ware, J.; Kosinski, M.; Bjorner, J.; Turner-Bowker, D.; Gandek, B.; Maruish, M. Development. In *User's Manual for the SF-36v2® Health Survey*, 2nd ed.; QualityMetric Incorporated: Johnston, RI, USA, 2007.
16. Taylor, R.S.; Dalal, H.; Jolly, K.; Moxham, T.; Zawada, A. Home-based versus center-based cardiac rehabilitation. *Cochrane Database Syst. Rev.* **2020**, *1*, CD007130. [CrossRef]
17. Shaw, L.J.; Bugiardini, R.; Merz, C.N.B. Women and ischemic heart disease: Evolving knowledge. *J. Am. Coll. Cardiol.* **2009**, *54*, 1561–1575. [CrossRef] [PubMed]
18. Grace, S.L.; Turk-Adawi, K.I.; Contractor, A.; Atrey, A.; Campbell, N.; Derman, W.; Ghisi, G.L.; Oldridge, N.; Sarkar, B.K.; Yeo, T.J.; et al. Cardiac rehabilitation delivery model for low-resource settings. *Heart* **2016**, *102*, 1449–1455. [CrossRef]
19. Artinian, N.T.; Abrams, J.; Keteyian, S.J.; Franks, M.M.; Franklin, B.; Pienta, A.; Tkatch, R.; Cuff, L.; Alexander, P.; Schwartz, S. Correlates of depression at baseline among African Americans enrolled in cardiac rehabilitation. *J. Cardiopulm. Rehabilit. Prev.* **2009**, *29*, 24–31. [CrossRef]
20. Anderson, L.; Oldridge, N.; Thompson, D.R.; Zwisler, A.D.; Rees, K.; Martin, N.; Taylor, R.S. Exercise-based cardiac rehabilitation for coronary heart disease: Cochrane systematic review and meta-analysis. *J. Am. Coll. Cardiol.* **2016**, *67*, 1–12. [CrossRef]
21. Pierucci, N.; Laviola, D.; Mariani, M.V.; Nardini, A.; Adamo, F.; Mahfouz, K.; Colaiaco, C.; Ammirati, F.; Santini, L.; Lavalle, C. Remote monitoring and heart failure. *Eur. Heart J. Suppl.* **2025**, *27*, i126–i131. [CrossRef] [PubMed] [PubMed Central]
22. Thomas, R.J.; Beatty, A.L.; Beckie, T.M.; Brewer, L.C.; Brown, T.M.; Forman, D.E.; Franklin, B.A.; Keteyian, S.J.; Kitzman, D.W.; Regensteiner, J.G.; et al. Home-based cardiac rehabilitation: A scientific statement from the American Association of Cardiovascular and Pulmonary Rehabilitation, the American Heart Association, and the American College of Cardiology. *Circulation* **2019**, *140*, e69–e89. [CrossRef]
23. Jin, K.; Khonsari, S.; Gallagher, R.; Gallagher, P.; Clark, A.M.; Freedman, B.; Briffa, T.; Bauman, A.; Redfern, J.; Neubeck, L. Telehealth interventions for the secondary prevention of coronary heart disease: A systematic review and meta-analysis. *Eur. J. Cardiovasc. Nurs.* **2019**, *4*, 260–271. [CrossRef] [PubMed]
24. Rawstorn, J.C.; Gant, N.; Direito, A.; Beckmann, C.; Maddison, R. Telehealth exercise-based cardiac rehabilitation: A systematic review and meta-analysis. *Heart* **2016**, *102*, 1183–1192. [CrossRef]

https://doi.org/10.3390/jcm15020694

Journal of
Clinical Medicine

MDPI

Article

The Impact of Selected Risk Factors on the Frequency of Cardiac Rehabilitation: Part I

Andrzej Kleinrok [1], Marlena Krawczyk-Suszek [2,*] and Beata Zams [3]

1 Faculty of Health Sciences, Vincent Pol University, 20-816 Lublin, Poland; a.kleinrok@wp.pl
2 Department of Physiotherapy, Medical College, University of Information Technology and Management, 35-225 Rzeszow, Poland
3 Institute of Humanities and Medicine, Academy of Zamosc, 22-400 Zamosc, Poland; bzams@interia.pl
* Correspondence: m.krawczyk.umlub@gmail.com

Abstract: Background/Objectives: Cardiac rehabilitation (CR) is the most important element in the process of returning patients to everyday functioning. The aim of the study was to compare the frequency of use of various forms of CR in terms of the occurrence of various risk factors in patients after acute coronary syndrome (ACS). **Methods**: The study was conducted in a group of 1600 patients after ACS across 4 time points: 3, 6, 12 months, and 5 years. Patients were classified into four groups: (1) patients who do not participate in any rehabilitation programme after hospital treatment (0 + 0); (2) patients participating in a sanatorium programme (0 + S); (3) patients participating in an outpatient programme (0 + A); (4) patients participating in both forms (A + S). The study retrospectively analysed patients' medical records for the following risk factors: smoking, hypertension, and obesity. The relationship between the four groups and the likelihood of undergoing a given form of rehabilitation was determined (Odds ratio [OR]; 95% confidence interval [CI]). Group matching in terms of gender and age was also applied using Propensity Score Matching (PSM). **Results:** Among those who did not undergo rehabilitation (0 + 0) 6 months after ACS, compared to the baseline groups, the most common were those who returned to smoking (OR = 3.42) and those with persistent obesity (OR = 3.69); after 5 years–individuals who reduced their obesity (OR = 4.86; after PSM: OR = 6.51). The highest chance of A + S rehabilitation was observed in the 3rd and 6th month in the group of people who quit smoking (OR = 7.60; OR = 6.04), after 6 months in the 'reduction in uncontrolled hypertension' group (OR = 11.44) and after 3 months in the 'Reduction in obesity (after PSM)' group (OR = 7.80). **Conclusions:** The most effective reduction in selected risk factors is reached by participation in sanatorium and ambulatory programmes (A + S).

Keywords: cardiac rehabilitation; heart attack; hypertension; obesity; smoking

1. Introduction

Rehabilitation is an integral part of patient treatment and, depending on the disease, the rehabilitation process has different priorities, with appropriate therapeutic methods taken into account. The implementation of the rehabilitation process also depends on the severity of the disease and the stage of its treatment, as well as on the patient's abilities and acceptance of the methods used. Knowledge of the course and consequences of the disease allows the goal of rehabilitation to be determined. However, the effectiveness of rehabilitation depends not only on the patient's commitment, but also on the professionalism of the staff. Knowledge of the mechanisms of action of the therapeutic methods used enables optimal selection of the components of the process and the order in which they are applied.

In order to achieve a good rehabilitation effect, it is necessary to use several of the methods mentioned. Such a broad and interdisciplinary approach to the rehabilitation process is called comprehensive (holistic) rehabilitation [1–5]. One form of rehabilitation is cardiac rehabilitation (CR), which is widely recognised as a method of treating patients. It is part of secondary prevention of coronary heart disease and is divided into three main phases. In the early phase (phase 1), patient mobilisation is used during acute hospitalisation. Phase 2 includes rehabilitation services traditionally provided on an outpatient basis. The main goal of this phase is to change the patient's health behaviours, modify risk factors (RF), and improve psychosocial well-being. Phase 3 involves the long-term maintenance of the lifestyle changes previously introduced by the patient [5,6].

Comprehensive cardiac rehabilitation (CCR) is a special type of rehabilitation that involves a multidisciplinary approach. CCR encompasses individual elements of comprehensive patient treatment, such as patient assessment, management and control of cardiovascular RF, promotion and awareness-raising of healthy physical activity, dietary advice, psychosocial and occupational support. Each of these elements of CCR is essential for public health—favourable rehabilitation outcomes, improved quality of life for patients, and optimal costs [5].

The most common indications for CCR are acute coronary syndrome (ACS), status after revascularisation procedures and status after surgical treatment of heart disease. CCR is also used in clinically evident coronary artery disease, the presence of strong RF, high cardiovascular risk, and heart failure [5].

In the holistic implementation of the CCR programme, identifying and eliminating risk factors (RFs) is extremely important. The five main RFs (hypertension, dyslipidaemia, overweight and obesity, diabetes and smoking) are responsible for 50% of cardiovascular diseases worldwide [7]. Therefore, 50% of all cases of cardiovascular disease (CVD) can be prevented by effectively eliminating the main RFs [7]. However, CVD significantly reduces patients' quality of life; hence, measures should be implemented in this area [8–10]. Effective treatment of hypertension in people aged 55–60 adds the most years without CVD, and quitting smoking adds the most years of life [7]. Combating risk factors is particularly important. An analysis of the 10-year risk of death or cardiovascular disease in a population of 1.5 million healthy people worldwide showed that the presence of risk factors (systolic blood pressure, non-HDL cholesterol, diabetes and smoking) accounts for 57.2% of cardiovascular disease cases in women and 52.6% in men, and for 22.2% and 19.2% of deaths, respectively [11].

For the patient, the main goals of rehabilitation are as follows: the removal of symptoms, the consequences of the disease and its causative factors, as well as the restoration of the patient's full or maximum possible physical, mental, social and professional fitness and enabling a return to independence through the restoration of fitness [12]. The basic condition for achieving positive rehabilitation results is cooperation between professional healthcare staff and the patient. Cooperation with the patient becomes effective when the patient has knowledge and understanding, which ensures their motivation [1,12,13].

According to the guidelines of the European Society of Cardiology (ESC), CR has been classified as a class IA method in the treatment of, among others, patients with ACS. Forms of CR may include outpatient intervention, rehabilitation in a sanatorium setting, and, according to the latest guidelines, may also be conducted in the form of telerehabilitation, with satisfactory therapeutic results [14]. Given the ageing population, varying percentages of ACS patients in different countries [15], the economic burden on national healthcare systems, and, above all, the high risk of recurrence, secondary prevention strategies are an important pillar of public health and quality of life for patients [16].

The aim of the study was to compare the frequency of use of different forms of CR in terms of the occurrence of various risk factors in patients after acute coronary syndrome.

2. Materials and Methods

2.1. Organisation of the Study

The retrospective analysis was conducted by medical records of 1600 patients admitted to the Cardiology Department of Provincial Hospital Pope John Paul II in Zamosc in 2017–2022. The authorities of the hospital and the University of Management and Administration gave consent to carry out the study. The study also received the positive opinion of the Commission on Ethics of Scientific Research of the University of Information Technology and Management in Rzeszow (No.2/2022). The reason for the admission was ACS diagnosed on the basis of chest pain, ECG teletransmission from ambulance and cardiological teleconsultation. The decision to admit a patient to the hospital, bypassing the nearest hospital, was made by the chief cardiologist on duty. The described system covered a population of 400,000 inhabitants.

2.2. Patients

The study included 1600 patients with ACS diagnosed on the basis of chest pain, ECG teletransmission from an ambulance, and cardiological teleconsultation. The majority of patients included in the study were men (69.7% of the total), with an average age of 58 ± 10 years. Most of the respondents lived in cities (54.0% of the total). Before ACS, most patients were in the working population (46.3%); after the disease, most retired (46.3%). Among the risk factors recorded, the majority of respondents had hypertension (56.3% of the total). In addition, smoking was recorded in 32.0% of the group, and the average BMI was 27.0 ± 3.8 kg/m^2, which indicates overweight. Detailed data are presented in Table 1.

Table 1. General characteristics of the group.

Variable [n (%)]	Total N = 1600 (100.0)	A + 0 N = 412 (25.8)	0 + S N = 415 (25.9)	A + S N = 343 (21.4)	0 + 0 N = 430 (26.9)	p
Gender (male)	1116 (69.7)	252 (61.2)	265 (63.9)	265 (77.3)	334 (77.4)	<0.0001
Age (years)	58.0 ± 10.0	57.5 ± 10.2	58.2 ± 11.0	56.8 ± 9.2	59.2 ± 9.3	<0.0001
Place of residence (city)	864 (54.0)	223 (54.1)	201 (48.4)	229 (66.8)	211 (49.1)	<0.0001
Marital status (married)	1250 (78.1)	281 (71.9)	313 (75.4)	259 (86.0)	361 (84.7)	<0.0001
Education (secondary or higher education)	718 (44.9)	169 (41.0)	192 (46.3)	169 (49.3)	188 (44.8)	0.1432
Employment status at the time of admission:						<0.0001
— Employed	741 (46.3)	168 (40.8)	205 (49.4)	158 (46.1)	210 (48.9)	
— Unemployed	43 (2.7)	18 (4.4)	11 (2.7)	10 (2.9)	4 (0.9)	
— Retired	546 (34.1)	125 (30.3)	152 (36.6)	100 (29.1)	163 (39.3)	
— Disabled	194 (12.1)	61 (14.8)	17 (4.1)	75 (21.9)	41 (9.5)	
— Unknown	76 (4.8)	40 (9.7)	30 (7.2)	0 (0.0)	6 (1.4)	

Table 1. *Cont.*

Variable [n (%)]	Total N = 1600 (100.0)	A + 0 N = 412 (25.8)	0 + S N = 415 (25.9)	A + S N = 343 (21.4)	0 + 0 N = 430 (26.9)	*p*
Current employment status:						
— Employed	496 (31.0)	137 (33.3)	145 (35.0)	115 (33.5)	99 (23.0)	
— Unemployed	36 (2.3)	15 (3.6)	8 (1.9)	11 (3.2)	2 (0.5)	<0.0001
— Retired	741 (46.3)	152 (36.9)	207 (49.9)	121 (35.3)	261 (60.7)	
— Disabled	261 (16.3)	79 (19.2)	42 (10.1)	90 (26.2)	50 (11.6)	
— Unknown	66 (4.1)	29 (7.0)	13 (3.1)	6 (1.8)	18 (4.2)	
The illness was the reason for taking retirement	86 (5.4)	25 (6.1)	29 (7.0)	6 (1.7)	26 (6.1)	<0.0001
Medical data. risk factors and comorbidities (upon discharge from the hospital) [M ± SD]						
Physical activity [min/week]	342.7 ± 437.8	336.2 ± 440.3	102.5 ± 64.7	788.6 ± 535.4	169.0 ± 83.9	<0.0001
BMI [kg/m^2]	27.0 ± 3.8	26.6 ± 3.6	26.2 ± 3.1	27.9 ± 4.1	27.4 ± 4.2	0.0158
Diabetes mellitus [n (%)]	332 (20.8)	77 (18.7)	132 (31.8)	51 (14.9)	72 (16.7)	<0.0001
Hypertension [n (%)]	901 (56.3)	238 (57.8)	228 (54.9)	199 (58.0)	236 (54.9)	0.1615
Systolic blood pressure [mmHg]	131 ± 18.1	131.1 ± 17.3	136.3 ± 17.2	124.8 ± 14.7	131.6 ± 26.3	<0.0001
Diastolic blood pressure [mmHg]	80.1 ± 24.6	81.6 ± 39.9	83.2 ± 9.3	75.4 ± 9.6	77.9 ± 11.8	<0.0001
Smoking [n (%)]:						
— **Yes**	512 (32.0)	140 (34.0)	138 (43.0)	111 (32.4)	123 (29.9)	
— **No**	938 (58.6)	240 (58.2)	268 (66.0)	143 (41.7)	287 (69.9)	<0.0001
— **Former smoker**	122 (7.6)	32 (7.8)	0 (0.0)	89 (25.9)	1 (0.2)	
Left Ventricular Ejection Fraction (LVEF) [%]	54.5 ± 9.5	53.3 ± 9.4	51.1 ± 7.9	59.4 ± 8.1	54.6 ± 12.2	<0.0001
Hyperlipidemia [n (%)]	680 (42.5)	185 (44.9)	265 (63.9)	45 (13.1)	185 (43.0)	<0.0001

A + 0—ambulatory rehabilitation; 0 + S—sanatorium programme; A + S—sanatorium and ambulatory; 0 + 0—without rehabilitation; *p*—*p* value X^2 Pearson test analysis of the relationship between 4 groups (forms of rehabilitation).

2.3. Hospital Treatment

All patients underwent coronary angiography and revascularisation (angioplasty or surgical coronary bypass). The procedure was performed immediately in the catheterisation lab within 12 h of the beginning of chest pain. After the procedure, patients were hospitalised in the Coronary Care Unit (CCU) for 24–48 h. In addition to the nursing and medical supervision, patients have been undergoing passive physiotherapy from the first day, to prevent the negative effects of immobilisation and self-service learning. Medically stable patients were transferred to the Cardiology Department or directly to the Cardiac Rehabilitation Department, where they stay for 5–7 days. During this period, the passive and active physical exercises were realised in 60 min sessions under the supervision of the physio-therapist. The size of loads corresponeded to the patients' performance and capabilities. The sessions were carried out twice a day, 7 days a week, individually and in groups. Patients received oral and written information about the disease, its symptoms, treatment, and appropriate responses to symptom onset, as well as physical activity and diet. This information was also provided to the patient's family members.

2.4. The Course of Treatment After Discharging from the Hospital

After discharge from the hospital, patients visited the cardiological outpatient department. During the visit, the health condition was assessed, and after checking for contraindications, the participation in CR programme at the cardiological sanatorium and/or at the outpatient (ambulatory) CR centre was proposed. After the patient's acceptance decision, the patient was referred for a non-invasive examination of cardiac function and arrhythmias, and for a sanatorium stay and/or outpatient rehabilitation. The referral describes the current health status, medications and risk factors for coronary artery disease.

2.5. Rehabilitation Programme After Hospital Treatment

Stay in the sanatorium. The sanatorium programme included a stay of 1–3 weeks. Interval physical exercises were adapted to the results of the exercise test. Health education was conducted with particular emphasis on risk factors and their reduction. Dietary advice was given, as well as gymnastic exercises were performed. Ambulatory programme. The programme included 26 two-hour sessions held over 12 weeks. Interval: 30–45 min of physical exercise sessions were gradually increased by adapting to pulse limit. General gymnastics in both programmes included: warm-up, conditioning, strength and endurance exercises, followed by calming and relaxation exercises, supplemented with breathing exercises. Health education and dietary counselling for patients and their families were conducted. The consultations with a psychologist were conducted at the patient's request or for medical necessity. A resuscitation course for patients' families was conducted.

2.6. Analysed Data

Patients' data were placed in records containing the date and course of hospital treatment, as well as their participation in the post-hospital CR programme. Sociodemographic and medical data were obtained from hospital and outpatient documentation. Medical data included the occurrence of hypertension, diabetes, BMI, smoking, dyslipidaemia, and everyday physical activity (Table 1). The obtained data were placed in an Excel database. Depending on the participation in various patient rehabilitation programmes patients population was divided into 4 groups: group 1—patient who do not participate in any rehabilitation programme after hospital treatment (0 + 0), group 2—patients participating in sanatorium programme (0 + S), group 3—patients participating in outpatient (ambulatory) programme (0 + A), group 4—patients participating in both programmes: ambulatory and sanatorium (A + S). Data on the frequency of use of individual forms of rehabilitation, presented in Table 2, were calculated relative to the number of respondents in each group. In the case of the variables 'Return to smoking addiction' and 'Reduction in obesity (BMI $\geq$ 30)', the Propensity Score Matching method was used in relation to gender and age. The data analysis included an assessment of the dependence of the frequency of use of a given form of rehabilitation between the four groups analysed.

2.7. Statistical Analysis

Quantitative data were presented as numbers and percentages, and quantitative data were presented using means and standard deviations (M $\pm$ SD). The analysis of linear relationships between variables was performed using the Chi-square Pearson test. The probability of occurrence of a factor was estimated by determining the odds ratio (OR) and 95% confidence interval (±95% Cl) based on the frequency of occurrence of the factor compared to the initial group.

In order to reduce errors arising from intergroup differences in studies and to correctly estimate the impact of the intervention, the Propensity Score Matching (PSM) method was used. In this method, non-experimental data allow for the estimation of the effect of the intervention by matching individuals who received the intervention CR to a group of patients who did not receive the intervention.

Statistical evaluation was performed using Statistica, version 13.3 (StatSoft Poland, Kraków, Poland).

3. Results

An analysis was conducted comparing a group of patients without rehabilitation with groups of patients receiving various forms of rehabilitation while accounting for risk factors. The frequency of individual rehabilitation forms was reported relative to the total number of respondents and the number of respondents in a given group. The aim of this analysis was to identify risk factors influencing participation in the CR programme. The verification included four consecutive time intervals, followed by a re-verification. In the smoking group, significant differences between groups were observed at each consecutive time interval ($p < 0.05$). In the first analysed period (3 months), ambulatory rehabilitation (A + 0; 34.0%) and sanatorium rehabilitation (0 + S; 33.2%) were used significantly more often among ACS patients. During this period, 28.6% of patients did not undergo any form of rehabilitation (0 + 0). In subsequent time intervals after 6 months, 12 months, and 5 years, 0 + S rehabilitation was consistently used significantly more often among patients, and both forms of rehabilitation—outpatient and sanatorium (A + S)—were used least often. The same trend was observed in the group of patients who returned to smoking (after matching the group using the PSM method), where 0 + S rehabilitation was used significantly more often, or no rehabilitation was used. In the group of people who quit smoking, the most common form of rehabilitation within 6 and 12 months was A + S, while after 3 months and after 5 years it was A + 0 (37.0% and 44.9%, respectively). Among patients with uncontrolled hypertension after 3 months, the most frequently used rehabilitation was A + 0 (38.4%) and 0 + S (24.1%). After 6 months, 35.4% of patients most often did not attend rehabilitation at all or used A + 0 (29.9%). After 12 months, 30.8% did not use rehabilitation, and 39.4% used 0 + S. After 5 years, most often patients participated in sanatorium rehabilitation (0 + S; 45.8%) or ambulatory rehabilitation (A + 0; 25.3%). In the group of patients who reduced uncontrolled hypertension at each time interval, the combined form of A + S or A + 0 rehabilitation was used significantly more often ($p < 0.0001$). Of the total number of patients studied, 20.1% had a BMI ≥ 30. In this group, two extreme patterns were most commonly observed—either the use of both forms of rehabilitation (A + S) or neither (0 + 0), with the exception of the period after 5 years. In contrast, among patients with persistent overweight, regardless of the time after ACS, significantly more often, both forms of rehabilitation were observed. In the group of patients who reduced obesity at each time interval, both forms of rehabilitation (A + S) were most commonly used, although after 12 months, the frequency of their use decreased. In contrast, after 12 months, A + 0 rehabilitation was used more frequently (30.3%). In the group after matching (PSM), A + S was more frequently used after 3, 6 months, and after 5 years, while after 12 months (47.4%), A + 0 was reported more frequently. Detailed data are presented in Table 2.

The impact of the analysed risk factors on participation in various forms of rehabilitation was assessed. People who returned to smoking addiction 3 months after ACS were twice as likely not to undergo rehabilitation compared to the group of smokers (OR = 1.96), and almost 3.5 times more likely after 6 months (OR = 3.42). After a period of 5 years, the rates of rehabilitation use (OR = 1.05) were similar in both groups. Those who returned to smoking were almost 1.5 times more likely to use sanatorium rehabilitation 3 months after ACS (OR = 1.55) compared to smokers. No significant differences were noted in other forms of rehabilitation. On the other hand, people who quit smoking were more than 7.5 times (OR = 7.60) more likely to use A + S rehabilitation after 3 months, 6 times (OR = 6.04) more likely after 6 months, and almost 3 times (OR = 2.75) more likely after 12 months. Patients with uncontrolled hypertension were about 3 times more likely after 6 (OR = 3.42) and 12 (OR = 2.75) months not to use any form of rehabilitation compared to other people with hypertension. In the group of patients with reduced hypertension, after 6 months, the use of both forms of rehabilitation (A + S) was more than 11 times more frequent compared to the 0 + 0 group (OR = 11.44) after 6 months, 7 times more often (OR = 7.40) after 12 months, and almost 5 times more often (OR = 4.91) after 5 years. Patients who remained overweight after 3 (OR = 2.08) and 12 (OR = 2.40) months were twice as likely not to use rehabilitation compared to the obese group, and after 6 months, almost four times more likely (OR = 3.69). A significantly higher likelihood of using rehabilitation in this group was observed 5 years after ACS. Patients with persistent overweight were more than five times (OR = 5.36) more likely to use 0 + S and 3 times (OR = 3.15) more likely to use A + S than the group of patients not using rehabilitation (0 + 0). People who reduced their obesity after 5 years were more than five times more likely not to use any form of rehabilitation (OR = 4.86) compared to people with obesity. In this group, A + S rehabilitation was used three times more often after 3 months (OR = 3.10), five times more often after 6 months (OR = 5.22) and almost three times more often after 12 months (OR = 2.77). In the group after PSM, the lack of rehabilitation 5 years after ACS was recorded 6 times more often compared to the remaining group of obese patients (OR = 6.51). In the group of patients after obesity reduction, 0 + S rehabilitation (OR = 2.04) was performed twice as often 3 months after the onset of the disease compared to the 0 + 0 group. A similar OR value was observed in the group of patients who underwent A + 0 rehabilitation (OR = 2.0) after 12 months. Patients after obesity reduction underwent A + S rehabilitation almost 8 times more often after 3 months (OR = 7.80), 4 times more often after 6 months (OR = 4.44) and 12 months (OR = 4.24). Detailed data are presented in Table 3.

Table 2. Risk factors in subsequent stages of assessment (3, 6, 12 months, and 5 years) in various forms of rehabilitation compared to the group without post-hospital rehabilitation.

Variables [n (%)]	Total N = 1600	A + 0 N = 412	0 + S N = 415	A + S N = 343	0 + 0 N = 430	p *
			Smoking			
Initially	512 (32.0) **	140 (34.0)	138 (33.2)	111 (32.4)	123 (28.6)	0.5600
After 3 months	334 (65.2) ***	93 (27.8)	120 (35.9)	36 (10.8)	85 (25.4)	<0.0001
After 6 months	250 (48.8) ***	59 (23.6)	83 (33.2)	33 (13.2)	75 (30.0)	<0.0001
After 12 months	354 (69.1) ***	94 (26.6)	112 (31.6)	57 (16.1)	91 (25.7)	0.0031
After 5 years	232 (45.3) ***	62 (26.7)	80 (34.5)	41 (17.7)	49 (21.1)	0.0082
Return to smoking addiction [after Propensity Score Matching (based on gender + age)]						
After 3 months	325 (63.5) ***	92 (28.3)	118 (36.3)	30 (9.2)	85 (26.2)	<0.0001
After 6 months	240 (46.9) ***	58 (24.2)	82 (34.2)	27 (11.3)	74 (30.8)	<0.0001
After 12 months	340 (66.4) ***	90 (26.5)	111 (32.6)	51 (15.0)	88 (25.9)	<0.0001
After 5 years	219 (42.8) ***	55 (25.1)	78 (35.6)	37 (16.9)	49 (22.4)	0.0005

Table 2. *Cont.*

Variables [n (%)]	Total N = 1600	A + 0 N = 412	0 + S N = 415	A + S N = 343	0 + 0 N = 430	p *
			Giving up smoking			
After 3 months	81 (15.8) ***	30 (37.0)	11 (13.6)	32 (39.5)	18 (22.2)	<0.0001
After 6 months	146 (28.5) ***	61 (41.8)	42 (28.8)	31 (21.2)	12 (8.2)	0.0008
After 12 months	80 (15.6) ***	39 (48.8)	15 (18.8)	19 (23.8)	7 (8.8)	0.0003
After 5 years	156 (30.5) ***	70 (44.9)	47 (30.1)	25 (16.0)	14 (9.0)	0.0709
			The occurrence of uncontrolled hypertension			
	Total N = 991	A + 0 N = 273	0 + S N = 266	A + S N = 343	0 + 0 N = 430	p *
Initially	505 (51.0) **	174 (34.5)	206 (40.8)	91 (18.0)	34 (6.7)	<0.0001
After 3 months	411 (81.4) ***	158 (38.4)	99 (24.1)	65 (15.8)	89 (21.7)	<0.0001
After 6 months	268 (53.1) ***	80 (29.9)	73 (27.2)	20 (7.5)	95 (35.4)	<0.0001
After 12 months	419 (83.0) ***	84 (20,0)	165 (39.4)	41 (9.8)	129 (30.8)	<0.0001
After 5 years	336 (66.5) ***	85 (25.3)	154 (45.8)	29 (8.6)	68 (20.2)	<0.0001
			Reduction in uncontrolled hypertension (systolic ≥140 or diastolic ≥90 mmHg) in patients with HA			
After 3 months	401 (40.5) **	115 (28.7)	55 (13.7)	143 (35.7)	88 (21.9)	<0.0001
After 6 months	539 (54.4) **	193 (35.8)	80 (14.8)	188 (34.9)	78 (14.5)	<0.0001
After 12 months	489 (49.3) **	169 (34.6)	92 (18.8)	160 (32.7)	68 (13.9)	<0.0001
After 5 years	346 (34.9) **	118 (34.1)	98 (28.3)	88 (25.4)	42 (12.1)	<0.0001
			Obesity (BMI ≥ 30)			
	Total N = 1600	A + 0 N = 412	0 + S N = 365	A + S N = 343	0 + 0 N = 234	p *
Initially	321 (20.1) ***	60 (18.7)	57 (17.8)	105 (32.7)	99 (30.8)	<0.0001
After 3 months	254 (79.1) ***	61 (24.0)	40 (15.7)	88 (34.6)	65 (25.6)	<0.0001
After 6 months	205 (63.9) ***	45 (22.0)	37 (18.0)	71 (34.6)	52 (25.4)	<0.0001
After 12 months	222 (69.2) ***	47 (21.2)	37 (16.7)	84 (37.8)	54 (24.3)	<0.0001
After 5 years	155 (48.3) ***	38 (24.5)	42 (27.1)	56 (36.1)	19 (12.3)	0.0058
			Persistent obesity (BMI ≥ 30)			
	Total N = 321	A + 0 N = 60	0 + S N = 57	A + S N = 105	0 + 0 N = 99	p *
After 3 months	241 (75.1) ***	55 (22.8)	40 (16.6)	84 (34.9)	62 (25.7)	0.0409
After 6 months	199 (62.0) ***	44 (22.1)	36 (18.1)	69 (34.7)	50 (25.1)	0.0003
After 12 months	191 (59.5) ***	37 (19.4)	35 (18.3)	68 (35.6)	51 (26.7)	0.0037
After 5 years	118 (36.8) ***	26 (22.0)	38 (32.2)	43 (36.4)	11 (9.3)	<0.0001
			Reduction of obesity (BMI ≥ 30)			
After 3 months	35 (10.9) ***	5 (14.3)	4 (11.4)	21 (60.0)	5 (14.3)	0.0409
After 6 months	60 (18.7) ***	16 (26.7)	3 (5.0)	36 (60.0)	6 (10.0)	0.0003
After 12 months	76 (23.7) ***	23 (30.3)	6 (7.9)	37 (48.7)	10 (13.2)	<0.0001
After 5 years	150 (46.7) ***	32 (21.3)	6 (4.0)	62 (41.3)	50 (33.3)	<0.0001

Table 2. *Cont.*

Variables [n (%)]	Total N = 1600	A + 0 N = 412	0 + S N = 415	A + S N = 343	0 + 0 N = 430	p *
Reduction of obesity (BMI ≥ 30) [after Propensity Score Matching (based on gender + age)]						
After 3 months	19 (5.9) ***	2 (10.5)	4 (21.2)	12 (63.2)	1 (5.3)	0.0202
After 6 months	30 (9.3) ***	10 (33.3)	2 (6.7)	16 (53.3)	2 (6.7)	0.0410
After 12 months	38 (11.8) ***	18 (47.4)	4 (10.5)	14 (36.8)	2 (5.3)	0.0124
After 5 years	73 (22.7) ***	23 (31.5)	3 (4.1)	27 (37.0)	20 (27.4)	<0.0001

A + 0—ambulatory rehabilitation; 0 + S—sanatorium programme; A + S—sanatorium and ambulatory; 0 + 0—without rehabilitation; p *—p value X^2 Pearson test analysis of the relationship between 4 groups (forms of rehabilitation); [n (%)]—percentage of the number of people in a given group [3, 6, 12 months, 5 years]; **—percentage of the total number of people; ***—percentage of the initial number of people.

Table 3. Intensity [Odds Ratio] of risk factors at subsequent stages of assessment (3, 6, 12 months and 5 years) across various forms of rehabilitation compared to the group without post-hospital rehabilitation.

Variables	0 + 0 [1] [OR (±95 CI)]	0 + S [2] [OR (±95 CI)]	A + 0 [2] [OR (±95 CI)]	A + S [2] [OR (±95 CI)]
Return to smoking addiction [after Propensity Score Matching (based on gender + age)]				
After 3 months	1.96 (1.20–3.20)	1.55 (1.20–4.83)	0.84 (0.33–1.03)	0.11 (0.06–0.21)
After 6 months	3.42 (2.12–5.53)	0.79 (0.59–1.05)	0.64 (0.15–0.70)	0.12 (0.06–0.26)
After 12 months	2.08 (1.25–3.48)	1.15 (0.82–1.60)	0.77 (0.63–0.93)	0.21 (0.12–0.39)
After 5 years	1.05 (0.68–1.60)	1.31 (1.01–1.69)	0.92 (0.77–1.09)	0.60 (0.34–1.04)
Giving up smoking				
After 3 months	0.96 (0.40–2.28)	0.54 (0.32–0.91)	0.96 (0.70–1.31)	7.60 (2.50–23.07)
After 6 months	0.42 (0.16–1.07)	1.22 (0.74–2.01)	1.38 (0.99–1.91)	6.04 (1.90–19.15)
After 12 months	0.75 (0.29–1.96)	0.74 (0.43–1.27)	1.22 (0.87–1.70)	2.75 (0.90–8.41)
After 5 years	0.73 (0.32–1.67)	0.96 (0.62–1.50)	1.23 (0.17–1.23)	1.59 (0.58–4.40)
The occurrence of uncontrolled hypertension				
After 3 months	1.02 (0.86–1.20)	1.33 (1.07–1.66)	1.10 (0.87–1.26)	0.45 (0.30–0.68)
After 6 months	3.42 (2.29–4.59)	0.86 (0.69–1.08)	0.70 (0.61–0.80)	0.09 (0.05–0.15)
After 12 months	2.75 (1.98–3.83)	0.97 (0.80–1.18)	0.64 (0.56–0.73)	0.13 (0.08–0.21)
After 5 years	1.83 (1.21–2.79)	0.98 (0.78–1.25)	0.76 (0.65–0.89)	0.20 (0.11–0.36)
Reduction of uncontrolled hypertension (systolic ≥140 or diastolic ≥90 mmHg) in patients with HA				
After 3 months	0.98 (0.82–1.24)	0.75 (0.60–0.94)	0.90 (0.79–1.02)	2.22 (1.47–3.38)
After 6 months	0.31 (0.22–0.44)	1.16 (0.93–1.44)	1.43 (1.25–1.64)	11.44 (6.59–19.90)
After 12 months	0.36 (0.26–0.51)	1.03 (0.85–1.25)	1.56 (1.37–1.78)	7.40 (4.70–11.45)
After 5 years	0.54 (0.36–0.83)	1.01 (0.80–1.28)	1.31 (1.12–1.54)	4.91 (2.77–8.71)
Persistent obesity (BMI ≥ 30)				
After 3 months	2.08 (0.78–5.61)	0.90 (0.45–1.80)	0.96 (0.62–1.48)	0.32 (0.11–0.91)
After 6 months	3.69 (1.39–9.78)	1.09 (0.51–2.33)	0.65 (0.45–0.94)	0.19 (0.07–0.53)
After 12 months	2.40 (1.10–5.05)	1.07 (0.61–1.87)	0.68 (0.51–0.90)	0.36 (0.16–0.80)
After 5 years	0.21 (0.10–1.42)	5.36 (3.10–9.27)	1.54 (1.17–2.05)	3.15 (1.46–6.78)

Table 3. *Cont.*

Variables	0 + 0 [1] [OR (±95 CI)]	0 + S [2] [OR (±95 CI)]	A + 0 [2] [OR (±95 CI)]	A + S [2] [OR (±95 CI)]
Reduction of obesity (BMI ≥ 30)				
After 3 months	0.48 (0.18–1.30)	1.11 (0.56–2.23)	1.04 (0.67–1.60)	3.10 (1.10–8.74)
After 6 months	0.27 (0.10–0.72)	0.91 (0.43–1.95)	1.54 (1.07–1.21)	5.22 (1.90–14.35)
After 12 months	0.42 (0.20–0.87)	0.93 (0.56–1.63)	1.47 (1.10–1.96)	2.77 (1.25–6.13)
After 5 years	4.86 (2.39–9.90)	0.19 (0.11–0.32)	0.65 (0.49–0.86)	0.32 (0.15–0.68)
Reduction of obesity (BMI ≥ 30) [after Propensity Score Matching (based on gender + age)]				
After 3 months	0.23 (0.03–1.82)	2.04 (0.64–6.48)	1.07 (0.47–2.47)	7.80 (0.92–65.90)
After 6 months	0.34 (0.07–1.54)	0.91 (0.32–2.61)	1.43 (0.83–2.48)	4.44 (0.90–21.93)
After 12 months	0.21 (0.05–0.94)	1.44 (0.58–3.63)	2.00 (1.17–3.40)	4.24 (0.86–20.90)
After 5 years	6.51 (2.08–20.39)	0.16 (0.07–0.35)	0.62 (0.41–0.95)	0.22 (0.06–0.73)

A + 0—ambulatory rehabilitation; 0 + S—sanatorium programme; A + S—sanatorium and ambulatory; 0 + 0—without rehabilitation; OR—Odds Ratio; ±95 CI—95% confidence interval; [1]—relative to: the remaining group with uncontrolled hypertension [for the analysis of hypertension], the remaining group of initial smokers [for the analysis of smoking], the remaining group with obesity [for the analysis of obesity]; [2]—relative to group 0 + 0.

4. Discussion

The benefits of CCR are widely recognised. They can be divided into physiological, anatomical, psychological, epidemiological and economic benefits [5,17,18]. CCR is based on physical training and modification or elimination of RF (smoking addiction, lipid disorders, body weight, blood pressure, etc.) [19]. Hence, the authors included smoking, hypertension, and obesity in their analysis as factors modifying participation in CR. The most important benefits of CCR include a 26% reduction in cardiovascular mortality, a 23% reduction in hospitalisation rates, an 18% reduction in recurrent heart attacks, as well as an improvement in quality of life and a reduction in treatment costs [19].

The CCR process can be carried out in a hospital, an outpatient clinic, a sanatorium, or at the patient's home, depending on the patient's goals, capabilities, and preferences. The CR process can be divided into three [13,18] or four stages [4]. Both divisions are similar in terms of their goals and methods of implementation. The entire CCR process can also be divided into hospital and post-hospital parts. The post-hospital part of CCR can be divided into two periods: an active, organised period carried out in a sanatorium or outpatient CCR centre, and a passive, unorganised period in which the patient follows the principles of a healthy lifestyle individually or in groups.

The first stage of CCR is carried out during the patient's stay in the hospital. It applies to patients in the acute phase of the disease. It takes place in Coronary Care Units (CCUs), Post-Operative Wards, Cardiac Rehabilitation Wards or specialist hospital wards. The implementation of the CR programme in the acute phase of the disease results in a reduction in hospitalisation time, mortality, and the need for repeat revascularisation procedures [4]. The aim of the first stage is to help the patient achieve independence in everyday life as quickly as possible, counteract the effects of immobilisation and provide basic knowledge about the disease, its consequences and RF. In recent decades, there has been a systematic reduction in the length of hospitalisation for patients with ACS. Patients treated invasively with coronary angioplasty are discharged from the hospital within 4–7 days, provided there are no complications. For these reasons, the CR hospital programme for these patients is more informative than therapeutic in nature. The prerequisite for achieving the set goals is the implementation of CCR [4,5].

The second stage is carried out at home, in a sanatorium and/or in an outpatient centre. The patient's place of residence is a common location for the second stage. Such a location for the rehabilitation process is usually limited in scope, without supervision or the possibility of correction, and is not very effective. A more effective CCR option is to participate in a CCR programme at a sanatorium, an outpatient centre, or both, due to the possibility of active interaction and cooperation between the patient and medical staff and the provision of appropriate motivation and healthy habits. An important goal of the second stage is to implement a healthy lifestyle through education on combating RF, mainly smoking, blood pressure control, weight reduction, reduction of emotional tension, and reduction of the sense of threat, which leads to an improvement in quality of life [3,17,18,20].

CCR programmes in Europe usually last between 2 and 24 weeks, while in the USA, they last between 6 and 36 weeks [4]. A comparison of the effectiveness of CCR in reducing blood pressure showed that longer programmes were more effective [21]. In the current study, we did not analyse the duration of rehabilitation, but the combination of A + S rehabilitation, which resulted in a longer duration of rehabilitation attendance, and in the group of patients with reduced uncontrolled hypertension, the chances of undergoing both forms of rehabilitation were 11 times higher (OR = 11.44) in this group compared to the initial group. This confirms that the reduction in hypertension was the result of several forms of rehabilitation, which were associated with a longer duration of rehabilitation. However, duration strengthens the patient's motivation.

The implementation of stage II in an organised form results in an improvement in prognosis, as assessed by hard points. In a group of patients after myocardial infarction participating in an outpatient rehabilitation programme, a reduction in the incidence of MACE (Major Adverse Cardiac Events) was demonstrated, along with reductions in lipid concentrations and BMI and an increase in left ventricular ejection fraction (EF) [22]. A meta-analysis of 31 studies involving nearly 230,000 patients after ACS showed a beneficial effect of CCR on all-cause mortality (HR in the prospective analysis was 0.37 and OR 0.20, and in the retrospective analysis, HR was 0.64) [23]. In turn, a meta-analysis of 85 randomised studies involving nearly 23,000 patients after myocardial infarction showed a 26% reduction in annual cardiovascular mortality, a 23% reduction in hospitalisations, an 18% reduction in recurrent myocardial infarctions [4,19] and an improvement in quality of life [24].

International research conducted as part of the INTERASPIRE project shows that CR is recommended to an average of 34.4% of patients, while in Poland, this percentage was 69.6%. Only 19.6% of the patients surveyed participated in $\geq$50% of the sessions, which was likely strongly associated with the final outcomes of rehabilitation. Furthermore, this percentage was associated with a lower incidence of persistent smoking and lack of physical activity, better control of blood pressure and LDL cholesterol levels, and more frequent use of cardioprotective drugs [16].

In the current study, we compared four different CR regimens, and thus different forms such as outpatient and sanatorium rehabilitation. The research indicates a greater likelihood of conducting A + S rehabilitation in individual groups of patients with risk factors than in the initial groups, or of not receiving rehabilitation, compared to other people who do not attend rehabilitation (0 + 0). However, in the case of A + 0 and 0 + S rehabilitation, no significant differences were observed, except among individuals with persistent obesity. In this group, there was a 5-fold higher likelihood (OR = 5.36) of participating in A + 0 rehabilitation compared with the group with obesity.

According to research, multi-component rehabilitation programmes produce better therapeutic effects than single forms of treatment [25,26], which is why A + S rehabilitation was included among the rehabilitation programmes in our studies. We showed a significant frequency of use of this combined rehabilitation in a group of patients quitting smoking, where the chance of using this rehabilitation regimen was more than seven times higher compared to those not using rehabilitation (0 + 0) after 3 months (OR = 7.60) from ACS and six times higher after 6 months (OR = 6.04). The longer the time since ACS, the lower the chance of using rehabilitation. This trend was observed in each of the analysed risk factor groups, except for persistent obesity (BMI $\geq$ 30). In this group, 5 years after ACS, the chance of participating in A + S rehabilitation was more than 3 times higher (OR = 3.15) compared to the remaining group of obese individuals.

CR is a class 1 recommendation according to available and applicable guidelines, but according to available data, it is rarely recommended to patients in European countries, as shown in EUROASPIRE studies [27,28]. Therefore, it is important for national cardiology societies to take action to emphasise the importance of CR in the comprehensive treatment and rehabilitation of patients after ACS.

The current studies form the basis for further extensive analyses assessing the severity of risk factors in a group of patients with cardiovascular diseases and their impact on patients' quality of life.

Limitation

The first part of the analysis allowed for the assessment of the feasibility of conducting specific forms of rehabilitation for a group of patients, taking into account various risk factors. It did not include a detailed analysis of ACS risk factors for specific types of CR. Their inclusion in the analyses will allow a detailed assessment of how the type of rehabilitation used affected the level of individual risk factor parameters. Therefore, in the next parts of the analysis, the authors will present a detailed analysis of systolic blood pressure levels, an analysis of average BMI values, an analysis of MET (Metabolic Equivalent of Task)—average energy expenditure during everyday activities by patients participating in this study and differences between females and males.

5. Conclusions

The conclusion of this study is that cardiac rehabilitation has a positive effect on some risk factors in short- and long-term observation. The therapeutic effect is influenced by the type of rehabilitation used, indicating that an outpatient cardiac rehabilitation programme appears to be more effective than one delivered in a sanatorium. The factors that contributed to an increased likelihood of participation in A + S rehabilitation, especially in the period 3 and 6 months after ACS, were: smoking cessation, reduction of uncontrolled hypertension, and reduction of obesity (BMI $\geq$ 30). However, the best results of CR are reached by participation in both sanatorium and ambulatory programmes.

Author Contributions: Conceptualisation. A.K.; methodology. A.K.; formal analysis. M.K.-S.; investigation. B.Z.; data curation. B.Z.; writing—original draft preparation. A.K. and M.K.-S.; supervision. A.K. All authors have read and agreed to the published version of the manuscript.

Funding: This research received no external funding.

Institutional Review Board Statement: A positive opinion was obtained from the Commission on Ethics of Scientific Research of the University of Information Technology and Management in Rzeszow (No.2/2022; Approval Date: 25 April 2022).

Informed Consent Statement: Informed consent was obtained from all subjects involved in the study.

Data Availability Statement: Data will be available upon request.

Conflicts of Interest: The authors declare no conflicts of interest.

Abbreviations

The following abbreviations are used in this manuscript:

ACS	Acute coronary syndrome
BMI	Body mass index
CR	Cardiac rehabilitation
CCR	Comprehensive cardiac rehabilitation
CCU	Coronary care unit
HA	Heart attack
HDL	High-density lipoprotein
LDL	Low-density lipoprotein
Non-HDL	Non-high-density lipoprotein
MET	Metabolic Equivalent of Task
OR	Odds ratio
PSM	The propensity score matching
RF	Risk factor

References

1. Jette, A.M. Opening the Black Box of Rehabilitation Interventions. *Phys. Ther.* **2020**, *100*, 883–884. [CrossRef] [PubMed]
2. Brown, T.M.; Pack, Q.R.; Aberegg, E.; Brewer, L.C.; Ford, Y.R.; Forman, D.E.; Gathright, E.C.; Khadanga, S.; Ozemek, C.; Thomas, R.J. Core Components of Cardiac Rehabilitation Programs: 2024 Update: A Scientific Statement From the American Heart Association and the American Association of Cardiovascular and Pulmonary Rehabilitation. *Circulation* **2024**, *150*, e328–e347. [CrossRef] [PubMed]
3. Zhang, S.; Lin, Y. Advancements, challenges, and innovative strategies in cardiac rehabilitation for patients with acute myocardial infarction: A systematic review. *Curr. Probl. Cardiol.* **2025**, *50*, 102934. [CrossRef] [PubMed]
4. Aleksova, A.; Fluca, A.L.; Beltrami, A.P.; Dozio, E.; Sinagra, G.; Marketou, M.; Janjusevic, M. Part 1—Cardiac Rehabilitation After an Acute Myocardial Infarction: Four Phases of the Programme—Where Do We Stand? *J. Clin. Med.* **2025**, *14*, 1117. [CrossRef]
5. Ambrosetti, M.; Abreu, A.; Corrà, U.; Davos, C.H.; Hansen, D.; Frederix, I.; Iliou, M.C.; E Pedretti, R.F.; Schmid, J.-P.; Vigorito, C.; et al. Secondary prevention through comprehensive cardiovascular rehabilitation: From knowledge to implementation. 2020 update. A position paper from the Secondary Prevention and Rehabilitation Section of the European Association of Preventive Cardiology. *Eur. J. Prev. Cardiol.* **2021**, *28*, 460–495. [CrossRef]
6. Dalal, H.M.; Doherty, P.; Taylor, R.S. Cardiac rehabilitation. *BMJ* **2015**, *351*, h5000. [CrossRef]
7. Global Cardiovascular Risk Consortium. Global Effect of Cardiovascular Risk Factors on Lifetime Estimates. *N. Engl. J. Med.* **2025**, *393*, 125–138. [CrossRef]
8. Krawczyk-Suszek, M.; Gaweł, A.; Kleinrok, A. Ranking of diseases affecting the health-related quality of life of patients in Poland—A cross-sectional study. *Arch. Med. Sci.* **2024**, *20*, 1567–1578. [CrossRef]
9. Krawczyk-Suszek, M.; Gaweł, A.; Kleinrok, A. Correlation of gender with health related-quality of life of patients in 13 groups of disease in Poland. *Sci. Rep.* **2025**, *15*, 15277. [CrossRef]
10. Krawczyk-Suszek, M.; Gaweł, A.; Kleinrok, A. Correlation of ageing with Health related-quality of life of patients in 13 groups of disease in Poland. *Sci. Rep.* **2024**, *14*, 26404. [CrossRef]
11. Global Cardiovascular Risk Consortium. Global Effect of Modifiable Risk Factors on Cardiovascular Disease and Mortality. *N. Engl. J. Med.* **2023**, *389*, 1273–1285. [CrossRef] [PubMed]
12. Burn, J.P.S.; Wade, D.T.; Allcock, D.; Copstick, S.; Dunn, J.; Grist, G.; Husbands, E.; Laws, A.; Whitney, J. *Rehabilitation and Complex Disability Management in Specialist Nursing Homes and Other Residential Units: Guidance to Best Practice. A Report of the Working Party of the British Society of Physical and Rehabilitation Medicine*; The British Society for Physical & Rehabilitation Medicine: London, UK, 2024.
13. Tessler, J.; Ahmed, I.; Bordoni, B. *Cardiac Rehabilitation*; StatPearls: Treasure Island, FL, USA, 2025.
14. Bralewska, B.; Wykrota, J.; Kurpesa, M.; Kasprzak, J.D.; Cieślik-Guerra, U.; Wądołowska, E.; Rechciński, T. Cardiac Telerehabilitation After Acute Coronary Syndrome Ensures Similar Improvement in Exercise Capacity as Inpatient Rehabilitation, Regardless of the Age Profile of the Compared Groups. *J. Clin. Med.* **2025**, *14*, 3143. [CrossRef] [PubMed]
15. Institute for Health Metrics and Evaluation (IHME). *Global Burden of Disease 2021: Findings from the GBD 2021 Study*; IHME: Seattle, WA, USA, 2024.

16. Kotseva, K.; De Bacquer, D.; Jennings, C.; McEvoy, J.W.; Ryden, L.; Ray, K.K.; Lip, G.Y.H.; Erlund, I.; Ganly, S.; Vihervaara, T.; et al. Cardiac Rehabilitation in Patients with Coronary Heart Disease—Provision, Attendance, and Outcomes: Results from the INTERASPIRE Survey from Fourteen Countries Across Six WHO Regions. *Glob. Heart* **2025**, *20*, 75. [CrossRef]
17. Damluji, A.A.; Tomczak, C.R.; Hiser, S.; O'nEill, D.E.; Goyal, P.; Pack, Q.R.; Foulkes, S.J.; Brown, T.M.; Haykowsky, M.J.; Needham, D.M.; et al. Benefits of Cardiac Rehabilitation: Mechanisms to Restore Function and Clinical Impact. *Circ. Res.* **2025**, *137*, 255–272. [CrossRef]
18. Jegier, A.; Szalewska, D.; Mawlichanów, A.; Bednarczyk, T.; Eysymontt, Z.; Gałaszek, M.; Mamcarz, A.; Mierzyńska, A.; Piotrowicz, E.; Piotrowicz, R.; et al. Comprehensive cardiac rehabilitation as the keystone in the secondary prevention of cardiovascular disease. *Kardiol. Pol.* **2021**, *79*, 901–916. [CrossRef]
19. Dibben, G.; Faulkner, J.; Oldridge, N.; Rees, K.; Thompson, D.R.; Zwisler, A.-D.; Taylor, R.S. Exercise-based cardiac rehabilitation for coronary heart disease: A meta-analysis. *Eur. Heart J.* **2023**, *44*, 452–469. [CrossRef]
20. Thomas, R.J. Cardiac Rehabilitation—Challenges, Advances, and the Road Ahead. *N. Engl. J. Med.* **2024**, *390*, 830–841. [CrossRef]
21. Quindry, J.C.; McNamara, M.; Oser, C.; Fogle, C.M. Cardiac Rehabilitation and Resting Blood Pressure. *J. Cardiopulm. Rehabil. Prev.* **2022**, *42*, E23–E31. [CrossRef]
22. Xiao, M.; Li, Y.; Guan, X. Community-Based Physical Rehabilitation After Percutaneous Coronary Intervention for Acute Myocardial Infarction. *Tex. Heart Inst. J.* **2021**, *48*, e197103. [CrossRef]
23. Salzwedel, A.; Jensen, K.; Rauch, B.; Doherty, P.; Metzendorf, M.-I.; Hackbusch, M.; Völler, H.; Schmid, J.-P.; Davos, C.H. Effectiveness of comprehensive cardiac rehabilitation in coronary artery disease patients treated according to contemporary evidence based medicine: Update of the Cardiac Rehabilitation Outcome Study (CROS-II). *Eur. J. Prev. Cardiol.* **2020**, *27*, 1756–1774. [CrossRef]
24. Xuereb, R.; Xuereb, S.; Xuereb, R. A 69-year-old woman presenting with shortness of breath. *Heart* **2020**, *106*, 1637–1702. [CrossRef]
25. Dibben, G.; Faulkner, J.; Oldridge, N.; Rees, K.; Thompson, D.R.; Zwisler, A.-D.; Taylor, R.S. Exercise-based cardiac rehabilitation for coronary heart disease. *Cochrane Database Syst. Rev.* **2021**, *11*, CD001800. [CrossRef]
26. Blacher, J.; Olié, V.; Gabet, A.; Cinaud, A.; Tuppin, P.; Iliou, M.-C.; Grave, C. Two-year prognosis and cardiovascular disease prevention after acute coronary syndrome: The role of cardiac rehabilitation—A French nationwide study. *Eur. J. Prev. Cardiol.* **2024**, *31*, 1939–1947. [CrossRef]
27. Kotseva, K.; Wood, D.; De Bacquer, D. Determinants of participation and risk factor control according to attendance in cardiac rehabilitation programmes in coronary patients in Europe: EUROASPIRE IV survey. *Eur. J. Prev. Cardiol.* **2018**, *25*, 1242–1251. [CrossRef]
28. Kotseva, K.; Wood, D.; De Backer, G.; De Bacquer, D. Use and effects of cardiac rehabilitation in patients with coronary heart disease: Results from the EUROASPIRE III survey. *Eur. J. Prev. Cardiol.* **2013**, *20*, 817–826. [CrossRef]

Journal of
Clinical Medicine

MDPI

Review

Impact of Family Involvement in Cardiac Rehabilitation—Insights from a Literature Review

Gabriela Popescu [1,2], Alexandra Maştaleru [1,2,*], Andra Oancea [1,2], Alexandru-Dan Costache [1,2], Cristina Andreea Adam [1,2], Carmen Rîpă [3,4], Carmen Marinela Cumpăt [1,5] and Maria Magdalena Leon [1,2]

[1] Clinical Rehabilitation Hospital, 700661 Iasi, Romania; gabriela.popescu@umfiasi.ro (G.P.); andra.oancea@umfiasi.ro (A.O.); dan-alexandru.costache@umfiasi.ro (A.-D.C.); cristina-andreea_adam@umfiasi.ro (C.A.A.); marinela.cumpat@umfiasi.ro (C.M.C.); maria.leon@umfiasi.ro (M.M.L.)
[2] Department of Medical Specialties I, "Grigore T. Popa" University of Medicine and Pharmacy, 700115 Iasi, Romania
[3] Department of Microbiology, Faculty of Medicine, "Grigore T. Popa" University of Medicine and Pharmacy, Universitatii Street No. 16, 700115 Iasi, Romania; ripa.carmen@umfiasi.ro
[4] Department of Preventive Medicine and Interdisciplinarity, "Grigore T. Popa" University of Medicine and Pharmacy, Universitatii Street No. 16, 700115 Iasi, Romania
[5] Department of Medical Specialties III, "Grigore T. Popa" University of Medicine and Pharmacy, 700115 Iasi, Romania
* Correspondence: alexandra.mastaleru@umfiasi.ro

Abstract: Conventional medicine relies solely on the interaction between the doctor and the patient, not necessarily including the family in discussions about therapy and diagnosis. Nevertheless, recent research indicates that the presence of a family member during a doctor's visit improves both communication between the doctor and the patient, as well as the patient's understanding of information related to their health condition. Additionally, by adopting this approach, family members can better understand what obligations arise at this stage and the patient's needs. Studies have shown that collaboration with family members has significantly reduced mortality rate and improved their quality of life, as the family strengthened their confidence in their abilities by providing moral and emotional support. Even though family support and involvement seem to be very important, sometimes patients have reported that overly active family involvement becomes intrusive, as it violates their privacy and disrupts their autonomy. That is why it is important for family members directly involved in recovery to learn to respect the boundaries set by the patient. Both the patient and their family experience stressful moments during this recovery period, which necessitate their attention. The involvement of family members in the recovery process reduces their levels of anxiety and stress, as they can closely monitor the patient's progress. Additionally, integrating family members into the rehabilitation program can provide further benefits for the patient, as the presence of a family member leads to increased comfort and motivation.

Keywords: rehabilitation; cardiovascular disease; family; social; support

1. Introduction

Following hemodynamic stabilization, patients undergoing coronary artery bypass graft surgery, myocardial infarction, or heart transplant participate in a cardiovascular rehabilitation program. This program will help the patient return to their pre-surgery life by managing risk factors, implementing targeted physical exercises, and providing psychological support [1,2]. The recovery process for patients with cardiovascular pathology can be divided into 3 phases. These are individualized according to the type of surgery and associated pathologies. During the first few days following surgery, the patient undergoes an acute recovery process that often includes light walking, exercises performed in bed or by the bedside, psychotherapy, nutritional counseling, and educational sessions on improving their lifestyle and reintegrating into society. The following two phases involve more advanced weight-bearing, treadmill, or bicycle activities, as well as physiotherapy. The healing phase lasts about six months, and the post-healing phase follows after six months and lasts for the rest of the patient's life [3,4]. In addition to training to increase physical endurance, muscle strength, stability, and coordination, patients are instructed to give up unhealthy habits such as smoking and alcohol consumption, to reach an ideal weight, and to keep associated pathologies under observation. Furthermore, psychological intervention is crucial for cardiac patients because it improves long-term results by lowering stress, anxiety, and depression—all of which are risk factors for cardiovascular disease—and enhances adherence to the rehabilitation program [5,6]. Ambrosetti and his colleagues mention the importance of family integration in the cardiovascular rehabilitation programme and highlight the importance of psychological support from the family, but without specifying the influence on physical health or adherence to the rehabilitation programme [7].

Inevitably, the psychological well-being of patients is profoundly impacted following major surgery. Consequently, this affects the process of recuperation. Evidently, a significant number of patients encounter moments of worry upon commencing the rehabilitation program, as they harbor apprehension regarding potential difficulties during physical activity or possibly a reoccurrence of a cardiac event. Linked to this apprehension, depression arises, and the patient experiences poor appetite, fatigue, and lack of motivation [8]. Despite the positive impact of cardiovascular rehabilitation programs on mental well-being, not all patients attain a condition of balanced mental health [9]. For instance, individuals participating in a study carried out in Sydney, Australia, had an evaluation prior to being enrolled in a cardiovascular rehabilitation program. Out of 4784 patients, 18% received a diagnosis of moderate to severe depression, 28% experienced high levels of anxiety, and 13% manifested symptoms related to moderate-severe stress. By the conclusion of the program, a mere 9% of individuals afflicted with depression reported any improvement, while among those struggling with anxiety and stress, just 15% and 8%, respectively, achieved any improvement. This group of patients was more prone to discontinue their participation in the rehabilitation program. Heightened levels of anxiety and stress result in depression, while depression and stress in turn bring on anxiety [10].

These accumulating conditions compel the patient to withdraw from society, therefore heightening the probability of a cardiovascular incident recurring [8]. Family support is crucial in such circumstances and can drastically impact engagement in the rehabilitation program. Within this timeframe, patients often require assistance with daily domestic tasks, such as cooking, shopping, and cleaning. The family is the nearest and most suitable source to address these issues, therefore ensuring the patient's sense of security. Furthermore, family members can provide sincere moral encouragement both in the early stages of recuperation after surgery and during the later stages of rehabilitation. Moreover, the family can facilitate the efforts of reintegrating into society and achieving psychological rehabilitation [11,12].

Medical guidelines emphasise the importance of family involvement in cardiovascular rehabilitation programmes, but none of them clearly highlight the short- and long-term effects it can have. Therefore, this review aims to highlight both the positive and negative impacts of family involvement in the recovery process.

2. Materials and Methods

The purpose of this review is to evaluate the impact of family in the cardiovascular recovery process. The inclusion criteria for this review included studies that addressed the importance of family support in the cardiovascular recovery process, even if this was not the central theme of those articles. Articles that were not written in English and those that included participants under 18 years of age were excluded. We excluded review papers, abstracts, editorials, statements, comments, and conference papers. As search terms, we used the association between the following words: "family"/"relatives"/"social" and "support", "cardiovascular rehabilitation". These studies were selected based on their relevance to the review theme, focusing on studies with the theme we addressed as their main topic (Figure 1).

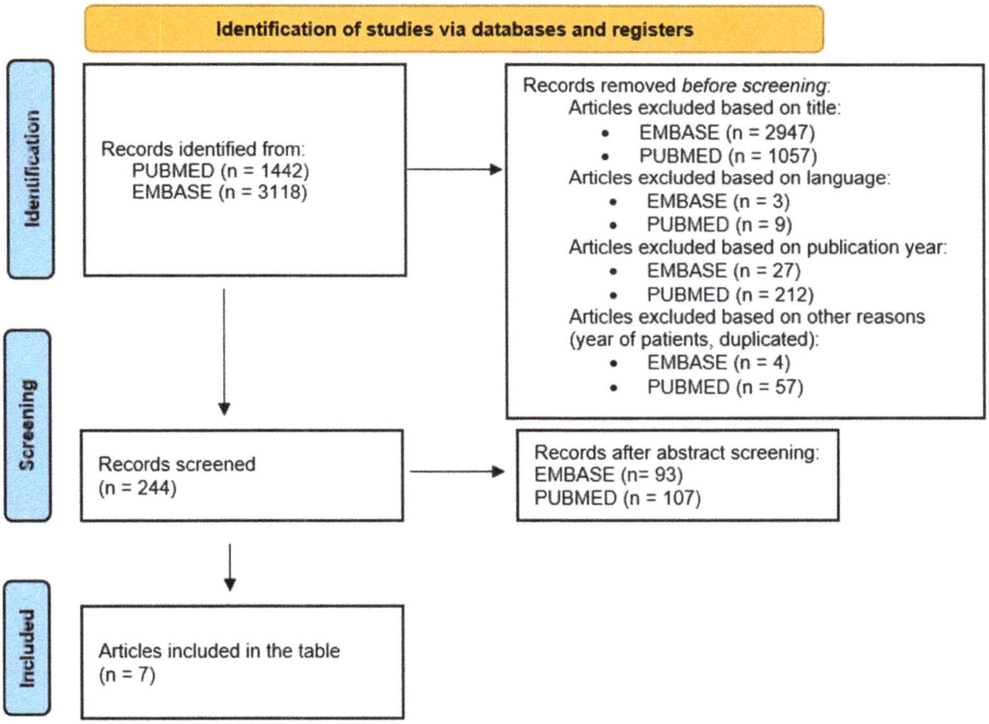

Figure 1. The selection process of the articles highlighting the importance of family involvement in cardiovascular rehabilitation.

3. Results

Although a broader body of literature addresses family involvement in cardiac rehabilitation, for the purpose of this review, we selected seven studies that we considered the most relevant and illustrative (Table 1). These articles synthesize the core evidence and perspectives on this subject, without claiming to represent an exhaustive list of all available publications.

Table 1. General data of included articles.

Year, Author and Country	Name of the Article	Number of Participants	Sex and Age of Participants	Patient's Diagnostic	Study Type
Vahedian-Azimi et al., 2024, Iran [13]	Cardiac Rehabilitation Using the Family-Centered Empowerment Model is Effective in Improving Long-term Mortality in Patients with Myocardial Infarction: A 10-year Follow-Up Randomized Clinical Trial	70 patients	61.40 ± 12.83 Years, 65.7% males.	Myocardial infarction	Randomized Clinical Trial
Zhang et al., 2024, China [14]	Clinical Effects of Hospital-Family Collaborative Cardiac Rehabilitation Training on Patients with Heart Failure after Cardiac Valve Prostheses	201 patients	Mean age 67 years, 61% males.	Heart failure	Retrospective study
Birtwistle et al., 2020, UK [15]	Family support for physical activity post-myocardial infarction: A qualitative study exploring the perceptions of cardiac rehabilitation practitioners	14 cardiac rehabilitation practitioners	No data available	Myocardial infarction	A qualitative study
Ma et al., 2024, China [16]	Needs and Constraints for Cardiac Rehabilitation Among Patients with Coronary Heart Disease Within a Community-Based Setting: A Study Based on Focus Group Interviews	11 patients	55–80 years, 72.72% females	Coronary heart disease	Semi-structured interview
Tuomisto et al., 2018, Finland [17]	Family Involvement in Rehabilitation: Coronary Artery Disease–patients' perspectives	169 patients	61–74 years, 76% males	Coronary artery disease	Descriptive cross-sectional study
Hagan et al., 2007, Australia [18]	Financial, family, and social factors impacting on cardiac rehabilitation attendance	10 patients	43–82 years, 80% males	Myocardial infarction	Semi-structured interview
Astin et al., 2008, UK [12]	Family support and cardiac rehabilitation: A comparative study of the experiences of South Asian and White-European patients and their carers living in the United Kingdom	65 patients	40–83 years, 55.38% males	Angina (32%), Myocardial infarction (42%), CABG surgery	Semi-structured interviews

4. Discussion

4.1. Does Family Support Matter in the Cardiovascular Recovery Process?

Conventional medicine relies exclusively on the doctor-patient interaction, without necessarily including the family in discussions regarding therapy and diagnostics. Nevertheless, recent research indicates that the presence of a family member during a doctor's visit enhances both good communication between the doctor and patient and improves comprehension of health-related information. Furthermore, by adopting this approach, family members can gain a deeper understanding of their obligations during this phase and the patient's requirements. This is particularly important, as several instances involve a lack of awareness regarding the gravity of the medical condition, leading family members to expect the patient to resume previous activities and habits promptly after the surgery [19,20]. Active family involvement is crucial for the patient. For instance, a significant number of individuals require someone to oversee the administration of medication, ensuring strict adherence to the allocated dosage and schedule. They feel let down when their children or close friends fail to demonstrate concern for their well-being [16]. Even so, it is crucial for the family to demonstrate understanding and avoid causing extra stress for the patient by consistently reminding them of the rules they must conform to [19,20].

Concerning family collaboration, males often have trouble expressing the adverse emotions that directly affect their lives after surgery. Conversely, women are more keenly impacted by the domestic chores they must manage. Unfortunately, it appears that in certain instances, women prioritize their household obligations above their involvement in the rehabilitation program and fail to provide time for hospital visits. Furthermore, research indicates that women who are currently employed or responsible for a spousal partner do not receive support from their families to engage in the rehabilitation program. Furthermore, for women belonging to ethnic minorities, collaborating with a man during the process of rehabilitation is regarded as religiously unacceptable [21,22].

Published in 2015, a study investigates whether a hybrid cardiac rehabilitation program, including family members, can enhance patients' quality of life by reducing the perceived stress and anxiety linked to a myocardial infarction in comparison to a conventional cardiac rehabilitation program. The study included a total of seventy patients with an average age of 61.40 ± 12.83 years, of which 35 were assigned to the intervention group and 35 to the control group. Out of the total, 65.7% were male, 98.6% were married, and they belonged to a family of around 5.37 ± 1.91 members. The caregiver's responsibilities included participating in all educational sessions with the patient, providing updates on the patient's home progress, and supervising the patient's activities during therapy sessions. The beneficence of this form of recovery was evaluated using six questionnaires that measured quality of life, health status, and depressive and anxiety status. In conclusion, the study revealed that patients who engaged in the rehabilitation program with their family members experienced more significant enhancements in their quality of life, physical well-being, and mental health compared to those who participated in the conventional cardiovascular rehabilitation program. Although there were no significant differences between the two groups, it seems that the support and optimistic atmosphere from the family resulted in both physical and physiological advantages [23].

In 2021, a study conducted interviews with 14 cardiovascular recovery practitioners to gather their perspectives on family involvement in the process. They stated that the family's presence at the doctor's appointment gave the patients peace of mind because there was another person with them who understood what the recovery process entailed. Very often, patients would come to the doctor demotivated and unwilling to engage in conversation, and in these cases, the family was a key intermediary. Moreover, in some cases, family members were actively involved in the recovery, trying to do the exercises and follow the rules, thus becoming a role model for the patient [15].

For a double-blind randomized trial at Shariati Hospital, 70 patients who experienced myocardial infarction were included, together with a small number of family members chosen by the patients. The purpose of the study was to compare the effectiveness of cardiovascular recovery with family members versus the effectiveness of conventional cardiovascular recovery. The follow-up period spanned a decade, from 2012 to 2023. The study participants selected individuals who were then allocated to participate in recovery stages 3 and 4, with phase 2 being entirely voluntary. Each patient and caregiver was provided with identical information regarding the exercises to be performed. Every group of patients adhered to a 2 h daily exercise regimen. Throughout the exercise sessions, family members assumed the responsibility of overseeing and providing guidance to the patient. Patient supervision in the control group was only carried out by the family, without any additional involvement. The study concluded that patients collaborating with family members significantly reduced their mortality rate, while the control group experienced a mortality rate four times higher. Furthermore, the patients expressed a favorable improvement in their quality of life, as the family bolstered their self-assurance in their own capabilities by providing moral and emotional assistance [13].

During an interview conducted by Natalie A. Hagan et al., patients expressed that the involvement of their family during the recovery phase influenced their decision-making process regarding lifestyle modifications and engagement in recovery program services. Although the family did not play a significant role in determining the outcome for some individuals, the provision of basic emotional support had a profound impact throughout this challenging time [18]. Additionally, a retrospective study published in 2024 highlights that a cardiovascular rehabilitation program based on collaboration between healthcare professionals and family improves the clinical outcomes of the rehabilitation program. Statistically significant results were observed, not only when evaluating patients' quality of life, but also in terms of echocardiographic parameters and laboratory tests [14]. In a cross-sectional study, six weeks after hospital discharge, 169 patients with coronary artery disease answered a questionnaire about their family's role in their cardiovascular recovery. Patients were asked whether their family helped or hindered them in the recovery process. Researchers wanted to know if the patient's family members helped with household chores, provided physical and moral support during the recovery process, and if they were interested in learning as much as possible about the patient's condition. Additionally, by using the questionnaire to analyze the harmful effects of such a serious illness on a family, the researchers aimed to determine whether the family experienced anxiety or depression during this period and whether their relationships deteriorated. Ultimately, the researchers concluded that most patients found genuine support in their families, and their relatives' positive and optimistic attitudes motivated them. Regrettably, this period has adversely impacted families psychologically and financially in certain instances, a situation that some patients have voiced concerns about [17].

When it comes to cardiovascular recovery, diet plays a crucial role, as an inadequate diet can lead to an increase in cardiovascular risk factors. Patients who have experienced a major cardiac event should limit their salt intake, stop consuming alcohol and ultra-processed foods, and incorporate more fruits, vegetables, whole grains, and fish into their daily diet [24]. It appears that the process of adopting a new diet varies depending on the patient's gender and their role within the family. In South Asia, the adoption of a new diet by a man often encourages the entire family to adapt to the new habits. On the other hand, women do not have the same advantage. In most cases, they cook for themselves and their family, and the pain and fatigue after surgery make them give up on a new diet and eat like everyone else. However, in some cases, the children take over meal preparation, easing the burden on the sick person [12].

Fortunately, in many cases, wives want to adopt the new lifestyle together with their partners. They prefer to take full responsibility for meal preparation and adhering to new habits, which motivates them and makes their partners much more optimistic when it comes to the recovery process [25].

4.2. Does Family Involvement Negatively Impact Cardiovascular Recovery?

Even though family support and involvement seem to be very important, sometimes patients have reported that overly active family involvement becomes intrusive, as it violates their privacy and disrupts their autonomy [15]. The patients express a strong desire to regain their independence promptly, which contradicts the families' inclination to provide them with maximum protection during the initial months after surgery, leading to conflicts between them [12]. Additionally, especially after the patient recovers from a myocardial infarction, the family tends to be very protective, affecting the patient's independence [15]. During an interview in a study, a patient reported that to protect him, his family started restricting him from leaving the house, intentionally creating distance between him and his friends. This social isolation, stemming from the desire to avoid another cardiac event, can emotionally affect the patient, leading to the opposite of the intended outcome [16].

Most patients with cardiovascular issues have unhealthy habits, such as alcohol consumption or smoking. After being discharged from the hospital, they receive a recommendation to give up these vices as they are among the main cardiovascular risk factors. Most of the time, the family puts pressure on the patient to give up these habits as quickly as possible, making them feel cornered and misunderstood. Even though giving up these two harmful vices is essential for cardiovascular recovery, the family should gently get involved in this process, as the patient will experience additional stress [26]. Furthermore, if the members of the patient's family who are directly involved in the rehabilitation process are not emotionally stable, they have the potential to negatively impact the patient's mood [27].

Fortunately, in many countries, there are national programs that help patients free of charge in their battle against addictions. These global and national programs to stop smoking and alcohol consumption provide free and accessible resources to support citizens in adopting a healthy lifestyle. In the United States, "Quitline" and the National Institute on Alcohol Abuse and Alcoholism provide counseling and treatment for quitting smoking and alcohol dependence. The United Kingdom and Australia offer similar programs, such as "NHS Smokefree" and "Quitline Australia," which include phone support, online resources, and treatment. In Romania, the Ministry of Health coordinates national programs for the prevention of smoking and alcohol dependence, providing counseling, medication treatment, and awareness campaigns. These initiatives reduce family pressure during the process of overcoming the addictions that patients had before the cardiac event [28–33]. In addition, over 70 countries have recently implemented restrictions on smoking in enclosed public spaces. Moreover, starting in 2023, at least 133 countries have raised tobacco taxes to reduce smoking rates and, implicitly, the increased number of illnesses and risk factors associated with smoking [34,35]. How family can negatively impact the cardiovascular recovery process can be seen in Figure 2.

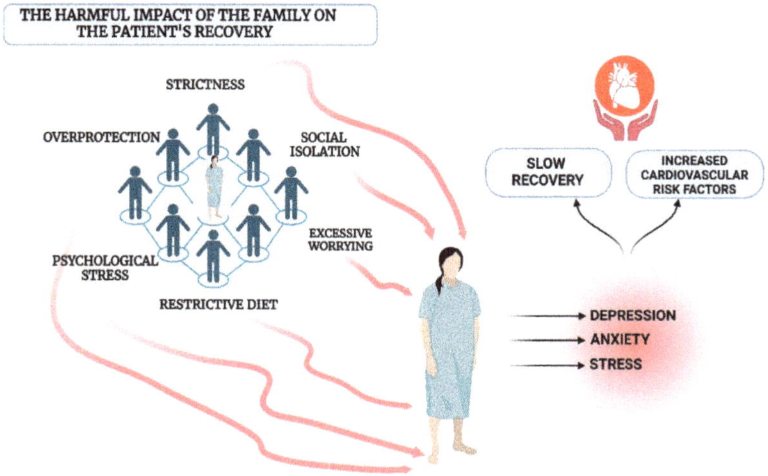

Figure 2. The harmful impact of the family on the patient's recovery process.

4.3. Does Involvement in Cardiovascular Rehabilitation Affect the Family?

During this recovery period, not only the patient but also their family go through stressful moments. The involvement of family members in the recovery process reduces their levels of anxiety and stress, as they can closely monitor the patient's progress. If the family is not well-informed about the patient's needs, instead of providing a positive contribution to their life, they can become an additional source of stress [15]. Following a significant cardiovascular event, the patient is unable to resume their prior lifestyle until they have completely recuperated. Consequently, the family experiences both the financial consequences and the responsibilities that often burden their spouses or children [17,18].

When it comes to changing their lifestyle, patients try to compel their close family members to follow the same way of life. In a study, a patient's husband recounts that most of the time he opts for a healthy diet just like her, but when he makes different choices from his wife, she criticizes him [25].

In general, when it comes to a rehabilitation program, the attention is entirely on the patient in question. Serious illnesses, such as cardiovascular disease, affect both the sufferer and their family. Patients' life partners, who are always by their side, experience the most stress. Family members' calmness improves the patient's mental state and accelerates recovery, as they are with them every day. When the patient experiences a catastrophic cardiovascular episode, undergoes surgery, and needs assistance, it impacts the family [27,36,37]. It appears that younger spouses are far more likely to have symptoms such as lack of appetite, sadness, and headaches than older wives. To observe the psychological and physical effects that occurred after their husbands went through a significant cardiac event, 213 spouses of patients who had experienced a myocardial infarction were recruited for the study. Following the completion of the psychological examination, it was determined that sixty-six percent of the participants met the criteria for increased psychological stress. Sleeplessness, a persistent feeling of tension, and emotional instability were among the most prominent symptoms experienced. The most significant stress factor (75%) was the thought that the treatment and rehabilitation program would not work, followed by the patient's emotional instability (66.7%). Younger age, the presence of minor children in the family, and a decrease in couple intimacy were the main factors that positively correlated with a higher level of stress among wives [27].

4.4. Socio-Economic Factors That Impact Cardiac Rehabilitation

Cardiovascular rehabilitation programs can provide cost savings of €30,500 per patient in the first year, mostly attributed to a resumption of employment, and up to €14,500 per year in the following years [38].

Despite the medical team's recommendations, statistics from the USA, UK, and Australia show that less than 50% of patients who have experienced a significant cardiac event follow a rehabilitation program after discharge. Analyzed data revealed a correlation between involvement in outpatient rehabilitation programs and advanced age, female gender, education level, socio-economic situation, the existence of comorbidities, and lifestyle [18,38].

The financial component is a prevailing concern among both the older and younger generations. Regrettably, as a result of increased expenses, several patients frequently opt not only to withdraw from the rehabilitation program but also to abandon the whole treatment plan, thereby removing drugs they deem insignificant [39]. Numerous studies have shown that the distance between the place of residence and the hospital might provide a significant challenge, particularly for persons living in rural areas or without companionship. Many patients prefer not to impose transportation concerns on their family members. As a result, in addition to medical service expenses, many patients face the challenge of transportation costs [13,18,38,39].

A crucial determinant in the choice to engage in rehabilitation programs within the financial domain is the level of job security. The majority of patients who are company owners consented to engage in a comprehensive rehabilitation program. Conversely, employed individuals attribute greater significance to returning to the workplace. The lack of comprehension among many companies about an extended medical absence causes anxiety among patients since financial security is a crucial factor for both themselves and their families. During the interviews, some patients expressed their intention to participate in a weekend-based rehabilitation program due to this issue. Despite all this, in the case of unemployed individuals, no increase in the participation rate has been observed [18].

The culture and environment of origin may also influence participation in cardiac rehabilitation programs. Individuals hailing from rural areas or belonging to ethnic minority groups often decline involvement in the rehabilitation program. Individuals frequently express a desire to participate in such initiatives within their local community, or they may outright decline based on their community's cultural values. Furthermore, a positive correlation exists between a limited degree of education and a low percentage of participation in these programs [39].

A study that investigated South Asian patients involved in cardiovascular rehabilitation programmes highlighted that family responsibilities usually depend on women. This situation leads to low adherence to the program because women choose to prioritise their duties as wives and mothers over their own health. The sociocultural environment they come from does not offer them support to participate in such programs; they believe that fulfilling family roles is more important than personal recovery. Additionally, several studies show that in Asian communities, time spent on recovery is perceived as a sacrifice made at the expense of the family. At the same time, Asian patients tend to attend consultations more often accompanied by children, which, combined with the language barrier, further complicates the recovery process [40]. On the other hand, patients of European origin more frequently benefit from the active support of their life partners, which is reflected in increased adherence to lifestyle changes. Thus, while Asian patients face difficulties in adopting a healthy diet, the families of European patients show a greater willingness to change their own lifestyles for the patient's well-being. Religion is also a determining factor, especially in the case of patients from South Asia, India, or African American communities, where religious and cultural norms can limit participation in certain recovery activities. For these patients, home-based cardiovascular rehabilitation programmes could be more helpful because they allow for easier overcoming of linguistic, cultural, and religious barriers [41]. In a different context, a study conducted in Brazil highlighted that the main reason for non-participation in cardiovascular rehabilitation programmes was related to family responsibilities, with patients not receiving family approval to take the time needed for recovery [42]. The majority of the time, patients are uninterested in cardiovascular rehabilitation because they believe that physical activity would further disrupt their health. Additionally, some patients believe that they get sufficient exercise while they take care of domestic duties [16]. When compared to the lifestyle they had before the event, a significant number of patients do not feel sufficiently motivated to embrace a new way of life [39]. Some studies have found that interacting with other patients who have experienced similar issues can motivate patients to adhere to the rehabilitation program. Moreover, group-based programs for patients and their interactions seem to help significantly anxious and depressed patients psychologically, as they feel much more understood when discussing their issues with someone who has gone through the same experiences as they have. In a study published in 2021, patients reported that team recovery motivated them to follow the program and made them much more positive about their long-term progress [43]. The high number of comorbidities associated with senior age makes participation difficult, even though retired patients have fewer duties and more spare time [38,43,44]. Furthermore, if the family does not prioritize the patient's recovery, they are less likely to be motivated to adhere [15]. Many patients seem to hesitate in making an immediate decision after surgery; instead, they prefer to return home to their families, consult with them, and only then make a decision regarding this matter [18].

When it comes to sex and gender, multiple studies have found that women have a significantly lesser presence than men. Frequently, medical personnel neglect the needs or the cultural norms of the community from which patients originate. It appears that strict weight and progress tracking have a substantial psychological influence on participants, causing them to decline involvement in group recovery programs [21,45]. Rehabilitation programs should be adapted not only to the patient's pathology but also to the participants' sex and gender since each has unique demands and requirements [21].

Furthermore, medical education is critical to the patient's engagement in the rehabilitation program. Doctors should not only focus on prescription medicine or recommending exercises for patients, but also actively engage in teaching, supporting, and instructing patients and their families about cardiovascular rehabilitation [16]. Regrettably, a significant number of patients choose not to engage in such programs due to the individuals involved. Patient feedback indicated that certain clinicians they interacted with lacked empathy and displayed excessive criticism. Additionally, the lack of a systematic arrangement to address the needs of all participants led them to abandon their efforts [21,46].

Hybrid programs that allow patients to participate from home, along with their families, are among the most feasible options today [13]. Patients who are included in family-involved cardiovascular rehabilitation programmes achieve good results in terms of symptom improvement, exercise tolerance, and quality of life. Thus, family support becomes essential for maintaining treatment adherence, monitoring symptoms, and continuing participation in programmes, thereby extending the impact of the recommendations in good practice guidelines [47]. Telemedicine is a more viable alternative, accessible even to patients residing at a considerable distance or having financial or cultural constraints that prevent them from accessing rehabilitation facilities [39]. The utilization of telerehabilitation enables the efficient monitoring of patients' physical training, particularly those diagnosed with cardiovascular illnesses, thereby facilitating sustained adherence to therapy without the necessity of hospital visits and the potential exposure to additional risks, including other infections. Based on its demonstrated safety, efficacy, and broad acceptance among patients with cardiovascular diseases, this strategy has great potential as a tool in the continuous battle against cardiovascular disease [48]. A summary of the factors that negatively influence participation in cardiac rehabilitation programmes can be seen in Figure 3.

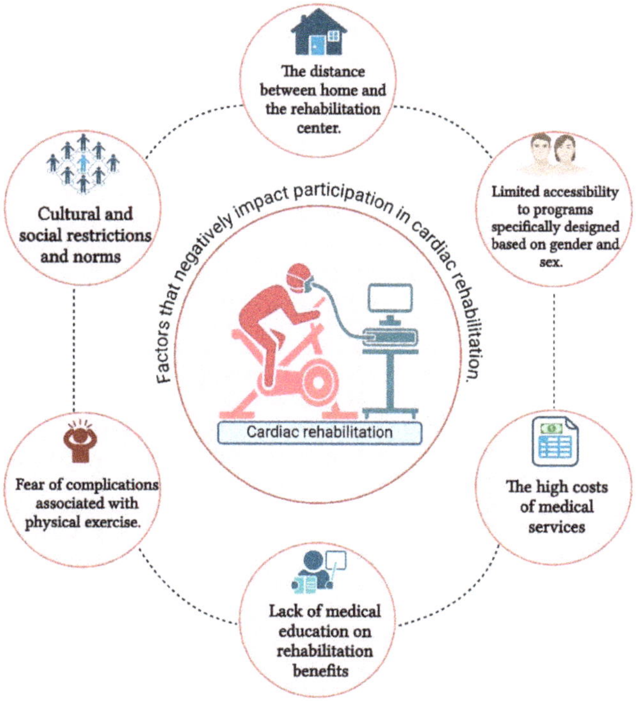

Figure 3. Factors that negatively impact participation in cardiac rehabilitation.

5. Conclusions

It is essential that family members, not just the multidisciplinary team, are integrated into cardiovascular rehabilitation programs, as family involvement helps patients acquire new knowledge and skills much more easily. Additionally, family can be a real help in reducing the patient's isolation. Family participation in stress management workshops or nutritional counselling, alongside the patient, promotes a unified approach to health. Thus, cardiac rehabilitation becomes a holistic process that not only provides professional guidance but also promotes active patient involvement and family support, improving engagement, well-being, and long-term outcomes [49].

Cardiovascular rehabilitation is a very important stage in the life of a person who has undergone a major cardiac event or is diagnosed with a severe cardiovascular disease. When a patient is enrolled in a recovery program, the physician should consider not only the pathology and the steps to be taken to improve the patient's health but also psycho-emotional and socioeconomic factors. Integrating family members into the rehabilitation program can provide several advantages for the patient since the presence of a family member leads to increased comfort and motivation.

Family members could be more sensitive to the cultural and social norms of the patient than healthcare professionals, resulting in a more comfortable setting for the patient. Furthermore, it would be more economically feasible to facilitate recovery at home, using telerehabilitation, but with the assistance of a family member. Family members directly involved in the patient's recovery must possess emotional stability, understand and respect the patient's privacy, and avoid imposing rigid constraints that could lead to long-term anxiety, depression, and social isolation.

A promising direction for optimizing cardiac rehabilitation programs would be the systematic integration of family members, not only through participation alongside the patient in certain stages of rehabilitation, but also through the development of structured educational programs specifically designed for families. These programs could serve as interactive learning spaces in which family members receive clear and tailored information regarding the objectives, stages, and benefits of cardiac rehabilitation, as well as their active role in supporting the patient. At the same time, such sessions would provide the necessary context for asking questions, clarifying uncertainties, and strengthening mutual trust between the patient, the family, and the healthcare team [50].

In the long term, the implementation of family-oriented guidelines would represent an essential tool for standardizing and harmonizing the information provided, ensuring access to scientifically validated knowledge. These guidelines could include detailed explanations about the structure of cardiac rehabilitation programs, the main clinical and paraclinical stages the patient undergoes, and concrete recommendations on how family members can contribute to treatment adherence, lifestyle modification, and sustained patient motivation. Furthermore, they could highlight practical strategies to ensure that family involvement does not create unnecessary pressure or conflicts, thereby preventing any negative impact on the patient–family relationship or on the emotional balance of both parties. Such an integrative approach would strengthen the family's role as an active partner in the therapeutic process, contributing not only to better clinical outcomes but also to improved patient quality of life and to a more balanced and sustainable family dynamic.

Author Contributions: Conceptualization, G.P. and M.M.L.; methodology, C.R. and C.M.C.; software, A.M.; validation, G.P., A.M. and A.O.; formal analysis, A.-D.C.; investigation, A.-D.C. and C.A.A.; resources, C.R.; data curation, A.-D.C.; writing—original draft preparation, C.M.C. and A.M.; writing—review and editing, A.O. and G.P.; visualization G.P.; supervision, M.M.L.; project administration, M.M.L.; All authors have read and agreed to the published version of the manuscript.

Funding: This research received no external funding.

Institutional Review Board Statement: Not applicable.

Informed Consent Statement: Not applicable.

Conflicts of Interest: The authors declare no conflicts of interest.

References

1. Patel, L.; Dhruve, R.; Keshvani, N.; Pandey, A. Role of exercise therapy and cardiac rehabilitation in heart failure. *Prog. Cardiovasc. Dis.* **2024**, *82*, 26–33. [CrossRef]
2. Balady, G.J.; Williams, M.A.; Ades, P.A.; Bittner, V.; Comoss, P.; Foody, J.M.; Franklin, B.; Sanderson, B.; Southard, D.; American Heart Association Exercise, Cardiac Rehabilitation, and Prevention Committee, the Council on Clinical Cardiology; et al. Core components of cardiac rehabilitation/secondary prevention programs: 2007 update: A scientific statement from the American Heart Association exercise, cardiac rehabilitation, and prevention committee, the council on clinical cardiology; the councils on cardiovascular nursing, epidemiology and prevention, and nutrition, physical activity, and metabolism; and the American Association of Cardiovascular and Pulmonary Rehabilitation. *Circulation* **2007**, *115*, 2675–2682.
3. Alexiev, A.; Terziev, A.; Gotcheva, N. Effects of an Early Cardiac Rehabilitation Following Heart Surgery in Patients over 70 Years. *SM J. Clin. Med.* **2017**, *3*, 1019.
4. Han, P.; Yu, H.; Xie, F.; Li, M.; Chen, X.; Yu, X.; Li, J.; Liu, X.; Shao, B.; Liu, J.; et al. Effects of early rehabilitation on functional outcomes in patients after coronary artery bypass graft surgery: A randomized controlled trial. *J. Int. Med. Res.* **2022**, *50*, 3000605221087031. [CrossRef] [PubMed]
5. Barbara, B.; Lin, T.; Greissinger, K.; Rottner, L.; Rillig, A.; Zimmerling, S. The Beneficial Effects of Cardiac Rehabilitation. *Adis J.* **2020**, *9*, 35–44. [CrossRef]
6. Wurst, R.; Kinkel, S.; Lin, J.; Goehner, W.; Fuchs, R. Promoting physical activity through a psychological group intervention in cardiac rehabilitation: A randomized controlled trial. *J. Behav. Med.* **2019**, *42*, 1104–1116. [CrossRef] [PubMed]
7. Ambrosetti, M.; Abreu, A.; Corrà, U.; Davos, C.H.; Hansen, D.; Frederix, I.; Iliou, M.C.; Pedretti, R.F.E.; Schmid, J.-P.; Vigorito, C.; et al. Secondary prevention through comprehensive cardiovascular rehabilitation: From knowledge to implementation. 2020 update. A position paper from the Secondary Prevention and Rehabilitation Section of the European Association of Preventive Cardiology. *Eur. J. Prev. Cardiol.* **2021**, *28*, 460–495. [CrossRef]
8. Gaffey, A.E.; Goldstein, C.M.; Hays, M.M.; Lee, S.Y.; Gaalema, D.E. Psychological Risk Factors in Cardiac Rehabilitation: Anxiety; Depression; Social Isolation; and Anger/Hostility. *J. Cardiopulm. Rehabil. Prev.* **2023**, *43*, E20–E21. [CrossRef]
9. Kowalewska, K.; Radecki, K.; Cieślik, B. Does Psychological State Influence the Physiological Response to Cardiac Rehabilitation in Older Adults? *Medicina* **2024**, *60*, 361. [CrossRef]
10. Rao, A.; Zecchin, R.; Newton, P.J.; Phillips, J.L.; DiGiacomo, M.; Denniss, A.R.; Hickman, L.D. The prevalence and impact of depression and anxiety in cardiac rehabilitation: A longitudinal cohort study. *Eur. J. Prev. Cardiol.* **2020**, *27*, 478–489. [CrossRef]
11. Barry, L.C.; Kasl, S.V.; Lichtman, J.; Vaccarino, V.; Krumholz, H.M. Social support and change in health-related quality of life 6 months after coronary artery bypass grafting. *J. Psychosom. Res.* **2006**, *60*, 185–193. [CrossRef] [PubMed]
12. Astin, F.; Atkin, K.; Darr, A. Family Support and Cardiac Rehabilitation: A Comparative Study of the Experiences of South Asian and White-European Patients and Their Carer's Living in the United Kingdom. *Eur. J. Cardiovasc. Nurs.* **2008**, *7*, 43–51. [CrossRef]
13. Vahedian-Azimi, A.; Sanjari, M.J.; Rahimi-Bashar, F.; Gohari-Mogadam, K.; Ouahrani, A.; Mustafa, E.M.M.; Hssain, A.A.; Sahebkar, A. Cardiac Rehabilitation Using the Family-Centered Empowerment Model is Effective in Improving Long-term Mortality in Patients with Myocardial Infarction: A 10-year Follow-Up Randomized Clinical Trial. *High Blood Press. Cardiovasc. Prev.* **2024**, *31*, 189–204. [CrossRef] [PubMed]
14. Zhang, L.; Wang, M.; Song, H. Clinical Effects of Hospital–Family Collaborative Cardiac Rehabilitation Training on Patients With Heart Failure After Cardiac Valve Prostheses. *HSF* **2024**, *27*, E1175–E1181. [CrossRef]
15. Birtwistle, S.B.; Jones, I.; Murphy, R.; Gee, I.; Watson, P.M. Family support for physical activity post-myocardial infarction: A qualitative study exploring the perceptions of cardiac rehabilitation practitioners. *Nurs. Health Sci.* **2021**, *23*, 227–236. [CrossRef]
16. Ma, L.-C.; Lou, S.-N.; Zhu, X.-L.; Zhang, R.-L.; Wu, L.; Xu, J.; Ding, X.-J.; Liu, J.; Wang, Y. Needs and Constraints for Cardiac Rehabilitation Among Patients with Coronary Heart Disease Within a Community-Based Setting: A Study Based on Focus Group Interviews. *Patient Prefer. Adherence* **2024**, *18*, 1141–1150. [CrossRef]
17. Tuomisto, S.; Koivula, M.; Åstedt-Kurki, P.; Helminen, M. Family involvement in rehabilitation: Coronary artery disease-patients' perspectives. *J. Clin. Nurs.* **2018**, *27*, 3020–3031. [CrossRef]
18. Hagan, N.A.; Botti, M.A.; Watts, R.J. Financial, family, and social factors impacting on cardiac rehabilitation attendance. *Heart Lung* **2007**, *36*, 105–113. [CrossRef] [PubMed]

19. Laidsaar-Powell, R.C.; Butow, P.N.; Bu, S.; Charles, C.; Gafni, A.; Lam, W.W.; Jansen, J.; McCaffery, K.J.; Shepherd, H.L.; Tattersall, M.H.; et al. Physician-patient-companion communication and decision-making: A systematic review of triadic medical consultations. *Patient Educ. Couns.* **2013**, *91*, 3–13. [CrossRef]
20. Koren, D.; Laidsaar-Powell, R.; Tilden, W.; Latt, M.; Butow, P. Health care providers' perceptions of family caregivers' involvement in consultations within a geriatric hospital setting. *Geriatr. Nurs.* **2018**, *39*, 419–427. [CrossRef]
21. Clark, A.M.; King-Shier, K.M.; Spaling, M.A.; Duncan, A.S.; Stone, J.A.; Jaglal, S.B.; Thompson, D.R.; Angus, J.E. Factors influencing participation in cardiac rehabilitation programmes after referral and initial attendance: Qualitative systematic review and meta-synthesis. *Clin. Rehabil.* **2013**, *27*, 948–959. [CrossRef]
22. Alsén, P.; Brink, E.; Persson, L.O. Patients' illness perception four months after a myocardial infarction. *J. Clin. Nurs.* **2008**, *17*, 25–33. [CrossRef]
23. Vahedian-Azimi, A.; Miller, A.C.; Hajiesmaieli, M.; Kangasniemi, M.; Alhani, F.; Jelvehmoghaddam, H.; Fathi, M.; Farzanegan, B.; Ardehali, S.H.; Hatamian, S.; et al. Cardiac rehabilitation using the Family Centered Empowerment Model versus home-based cardiac rehabilitation in patients with myocardial infarction:a randomised controlled trial. *Open Heart* **2016**, *3*, e000349. [CrossRef]
24. Kocanda, L.; Schumacher, T.L.; Plotnikoff, R.C.; Whatnall, M.C.; Fenwick, M.; Brown, L.J.; Rollo, M.E.; Jansson, A.; Burrows, T.L.; Duncan, M.J.; et al. Effectiveness and reporting of nutrition interventions in cardiac rehabilitation programmes: A systematic review. *Eur. J. Cardiovasc. Nurs.* **2023**, *22*, 1–12. [CrossRef] [PubMed]
25. Rowland, S.A.; Schumacher, K.L.; Leinen, D.D.; Phillips, B.G.; Schulz, P.S.; Yates, B.C. Couples' Experiences with Healthy Lifestyle Behaviors After Cardiac Rehabilitation. *J. Cardiopulm. Rehabil. Prev.* **2018**, *38*, 170–174. [CrossRef] [PubMed]
26. Borah N.; Bhawalkar, J.S.; Rathod, H.; Jadav, V.; Gangurde, S.; Johnson, S. Challenges to Cardiac Rehabilitation Post Coronary Artery Bypass Grafting: A Qualitative Study in Pune. *Cureus* **2023**, *15*, e35755. [CrossRef] [PubMed]
27. O'Farrell, P.; Murray, J.; Hotz, S.B. Psychologic distress among spouses of patients undergoing cardiac rehabilitation. *Heart Lung* **2000**, *29*, 97–104. [CrossRef] [PubMed]
28. Quit Smoking & Vaping: Get Expert Cessation Tips & Help Quit. Available online: https://www.quit.org.au/ (accessed on 30 August 2024).
29. NHK.UK. Quit smoking—Better Health. (n.d.). Available online: https://www.nhs.uk/better-health/quit-smoking/ (accessed on 30 August 2024).
30. Centers for Disease Control and Prevention. (n.d.-b). Available online: https://www.cdc.gov/tobacco/campaign/tips/quit-smoking/index.html/ (accessed on 30 August 2024).
31. United States Government. National Insitute on Alcohol Abuse and Alcoholism. (n.d.). Available online: https://www.niaaa.nih.gov (accessed on 30 August 2024).
32. Aliat, O.N.G. ALIAT-Asociatia Aliat Pentru Sanatate Mintala, (.2.0.2.4.; 30 June). Available online: https://aliat-ong.ro/ (accessed on 30 August 2024).
33. Ministerul Sănătății. (n.d.-b). Available online: https://www.ms.ro/ro (accessed on 30 August 2024).
34. More Countries Using Health Taxes and Laws to Protect Health. 2022. Available online: https://www.who.int/about/accountability/results/who-results-report-2022-mtr/more-countries-using-health-taxes-and-laws-to-protect-health (accessed on 30 August 2024).
35. Tobacconomics. Tobacco Tax Increases Around the World—August 2023 Update. (15 August 2023). Available online: https://www.tobacconomics.org/blog/tobacco-tax-increases-around-the-world-august-2023-update/ (accessed on 30 August 2024).
36. Van Horn, E.; Fleury, J.; Moore, S. Family interventions during the trajectory of recovery from cardiac event: An integrative literature review. *Heart Lung* **2002**, *31*, 186–198. [CrossRef] [PubMed]
37. Randall, G.; Molloy, G.J.; Steptoe, A. The impact of an acute cardiac event on the partners of patients: A systematic review. *Health Psychol. Rev.* **2009**, *3*, 1–84. [CrossRef]
38. Ruano-Ravina, A.; Pena-Gil, C.; Abu-Assi, E.; Raposeiras, S.; van 't Hof, A.; Meindersma, E.; Bossano Prescott, E.I.; González-Juanatey, J.R. Participation and adherence to cardiac rehabilitation programs. A systematic review. *Int. J. Cardiol.* **2016**, *223*, 436–443. [CrossRef]
39. Fernandez, R.S.; Davidson, P.; Griffiths, R. Cardiac rehabilitation coordinators' perceptions of patient-related barriers to implementing cardiac evidence-based guidelines. *J Cardiovasc. Nurs.* **2008**, *23*, 449–457. [CrossRef]
40. Ahmed, F.; Eberhardt, J.; van Wersch, A.; Ling, J. Cultural influences on adherence to cardiac rehabilitation programmes: Perspectives from South Asian healthcare professionals. *Int. J. Ther. Rehabil.* **2022**, *29*, 1–14. [CrossRef]
41. Carew Tofani, A.; Taylor, E.; Pritchard, I.; Jackson, J.; Xu, A.; Kotera, Y. Ethnic Minorities' Experiences of Cardiac Rehabilitation:A Scoping Review. *Healthcare* **2023**, *11*, 757. [CrossRef]
42. Ghisi, G.L.; dos Santos, R.Z.; Aranha, E.E.; Nunes, A.D.; Oh, P.; Benetti, M.; Grace, S.L. Perceptions of barriers to cardiac rehabilitation use in Brazil. *Vasc. Health Risk Manag.* **2013**, *9*, 485–491. [CrossRef]
43. McPhillips, R.; Capobianco, L.; Cooper, B.G.; Husain, Z.; Wells, A. Cardiac rehabilitation patients experiences and understanding of group metacognitive therapy: A qualitative study. *Open Heart* **2021**, *8*, e001708. [CrossRef]

44. van Engen-Verheul, M.; de Vries, H.; Kemps, H.; Kraaijenhagen, R.; de Keizer, N.; Peek, N. Cardiac rehabilitation uptake and its determinants in the Netherlands. *Eur. J. Prev. Cardiol.* **2013**, *20*, 349–356. [CrossRef] [PubMed]
45. Vishram, S.; Crosland, A.; Unsworth, J.; Long, S. Engaging women from South Asian communities in cardiac rehabilitation. *Br. J. Community Nurs.* **2007**, *12*, 13–18. [CrossRef] [PubMed]
46. Chauhan, U.; Baker, D.; Lester, H.; Edwards, R. Exploring uptake of cardiac rehabilitation in a minority ethnic population in England: A qualitative study. *Eur. J. Cardiovasc. Nurs.* **2010**, *9*, 68–74. [CrossRef] [PubMed]
47. Cersosimo, A.; Longo Elia, R.; Condello, F.; Colombo, F.; Pierucci, N.; Arabia, G.; Matteucci, A.; Metra, M.; Adamo, M.; Vizzardi, E.; et al. Cardiac rehabilitation in patients with atrial fibrillation. *Minerva Cardiol. Angiol.* **2025**, *73*, 13. [CrossRef]
48. Yang, Z.; Jia, X.; Li, J.; Mei, Z.; Yang, L.; Yan, C.; Han, Y. Efficacy and Safety of Hybrid Comprehensive Telerehabilitation (HCTR) for Cardiac Rehabilitation in Patients with Cardiovascular Disease: A Systematic Review and Meta-Analysis of Randomized Controlled Trials. *Occup. Ther. Int.* **2023**, *2023*, 5147805. [CrossRef] [PubMed]
49. Ghisi, G.L.M. Transforming patient education in cardiac rehabilitation: A vision for the future. *Patient Educ. Couns.* **2025**, *138*, 109176. [CrossRef] [PubMed]
50. Veloso, A.; Rocha, R.; Macedo, G.; Teixeira, A.; Almeida, V. Cardiovascular Rehabilitation: Perspectives of patients and healthcare professionals on the implementation of multidisciplinary programs. *Sci. Lett.* **2025**, *1*, 9. [CrossRef]

Journal of
Clinical Medicine

MDPI

Article

Randomized Trial: A Pilot Study Investigating the Effects of Transcendental Meditation and Yoga Through Retinal Microcirculation in Cardiac Rehabilitation

Adam Salon [1,2,3,*], Karin Schmid-Zalaudek [1], Bianca Steuber [1], Maximilian Elliot Rudlof [1], Till Olaf Bartel [1], Petra Mächler [4], Andreas Dorr [4], Rainer Picha [4], Per Morten Fredriksen [2], Benedicta Ngwenchi Nkeh-Chungag [5] and Nandu Goswami [1,6,*]

[1] Gravitational Physiology and Medicine Research Unit, Division of Physiology & Pathophysiology, Medical University of Graz, 8010 Graz, Austria
[2] Faculty of Applied Ecology, Agricultural Sciences and Biotechnology, Inland Norway University of Applied Sciences, 2624 Lillehammer, Norway
[3] Vascular Biology Center, Augusta University, Augusta, GA 30912, USA
[4] Rehabilitation Center for Cardiovascular Disease, 8061 St. Radegund, Austria
[5] Department of Biological and Environmental Sciences, Faculty of Health Sciences, Walter Sisulu University PBX1, Mthatha 5117, South Africa
[6] Center for Space and Aviation Health, College of Medicine, Mohammed Bin Rashid University of Medicine and Health Sciences, Dubai 505055, United Arab Emirates
* Correspondence: adam.salon.pro@gmail.com or asalon@augusta.edu (A.S.); nandu.goswami@medunigraz.at or nandu.goswami@dubaihealth.ae (N.G.); Tel.: +43-664-7924948 (A.S.)

Abstract: Background/Objectives: Cardiovascular diseases are a leading cause of death, and psychosocial stress is considered a contributing factor to these issues. With the rising number of heart surgeries, proper rehabilitation post-surgery is essential. Previous studies have demonstrated the positive impact of yoga and transcendental meditation on the cardiovascular system. This pilot study aimed to investigate the effects of yoga and transcendental meditation on retinal microcirculation in cardiac patients before (admission), after (discharge), and following (3 weeks after discharge) rehabilitation. **Methods**: This study examined changes in retinal microcirculation in three rehabilitation groups of patients after heart surgery. The control group received standard exercise therapy, while the meditation group incorporated 20 min of meditation, and the yoga group incorporated 20 min of yoga practice, twice per day for the duration of four weeks of rehabilitation. Retinal images were captured using a non-mydriatic digital retinal camera (Canon CR-2, Canon Medical Systems Europe B.V., Netherlands), and the microcirculation parameters central retinal artery equivalent, central retinal vein equivalent, and artery-to-vein ratio were analyzed using MONA REVA software ((version 2.1.1), VITO, Mol, Belgium). Repeated measures ANOVA was performed to evaluate differences between the three groups in the course of rehabilitation. **Results**: None of the parameters revealed significant differences in retinal microcirculation between the three rehabilitation groups. **Conclusions**: The study evaluating changes in retinal microcirculation, as an indicator of central circulation in cardiac patients undergoing rehabilitation, did not observe any significant changes. As yoga and meditation are underestimated approaches in cardiac rehabilitation, this pilot study acts as a basis for providing preliminary information for future studies to encourage the research community to fill the gap in this area.

Keywords: cardiac rehabilitation; exercise therapy; meditation; yoga; retinal imaging

1. Introduction

The review by Roth and colleagues, mapping the burden of cardiovascular diseases from the years 1990 to 2019, showed a continued elevation of cardiovascular mortality [1]. On 1 June 2022, the National Heart, Lung, and Blood Institute reported that each year, more than 2 million people worldwide undergo open-heart surgery [2]. The global improvement in healthcare is contributing to a growing population of elderly individuals, suggesting that these numbers may continue to rise in the future. Regarding complete recovery after heart surgery, an important part is played by a controlled rehabilitation program. There are different approaches to rehabilitation after heart surgery. They usually include exercising, emotional/psychological support, and lifestyle education to reduce the heart disease risk [3,4]. However, psychosocial stress and stress conditions are also associated with worsening cardiovascular health and should be prevented [5–7].

According to the International Yoga Federation, about 300 million people in the world practice yoga [8]. Among the major benefits of yoga are the enhancement of strength and flexibility, the improvement of respiratory and cardiovascular function, a reduced level of stress, and the improvement of sleeping and quality of life [9–12]. The National Institute of Health's national survey found that over 55% of yoga users report better sleep and that yoga reduces stress in over 85% of users [13].

Moreover, the estimate of people practicing meditation globally is between 200 and 500 million [14]. Data acquired between 2012 and 2017 show that the popularity of meditation is growing rapidly and has equaled the popularity of yoga, and it is highly likely that today it is already more popular than yoga itself [15]. It is a broadly known fact that even though yoga and meditation are related practices, they are not the same. While yoga involves physical postures, and breathing exercises, and can often include different meditation techniques, meditation itself focuses on mental concentration and mindfulness without physical movement and is practiced on its own, independently of yoga. The most common beneficial effects of meditation include improvement in negative mood and depression, a reduction in fatigue, the amelioration of blood pressure (BP) and lipid profiles, and a decrease in insulin resistance [16–18].

Therefore, the positive effects of meditation and yoga on mental and cardiovascular health are known [9–12,19–21]. While general meditation encompasses a variety of practices without a single prescribed method, transcendental meditation (TM) uses a specific mantra and follows a standardized technique. Previous research showed that yoga, as well as meditation, are effective approaches to cardiovascular health improvement, mostly decreasing heart rate (HR) and performing BP regulation. Other studies also confirmed the favorable effects of these practices on HR variability (HRV), anthropometric parameters, the lipid profile, and insulin resistance [18,22–24]. Several independent studies suggested that the mechanism responsible for this action is most probably hidden behind induced parasympathetic or reduced sympathetic activity after yoga or meditation [12,24–27].

The evaluation of retinal microvessel parameters is an innovative approach that enables the non-invasive and quick assessment cardiovascular health. This technique looks on the cardiovascular system through the parameters of small, repulsive arterioles and venules in the retina. The change in these parameters reflects modifications in retinal vessels. Previous research confirmed that these changes can reflect and predict future changes in the bigger vessels of the cardiovascular system [28–37]. Therefore, this technique is a promising approach with which to speed up the diagnosis and treatment of cardiovascular diseases. Data collection, as well as the verification of this methodology, is a big necessity in order to implement this approach to general practice.

Significant epidemiological and mechanistic investigations have shown that psychosocial stress plays a role in the development and clinical occurrence of cardiovascular disease

(CVD) [38]. The alleviation of psychosocial stress is considered one of the primary objectives in cardiac rehabilitation, alongside the promotion of physical activity and the enhancement of dietary habits [39]. Meditation and yoga represent two distinct approaches that can be employed to enhance mindfulness and alleviate stress and their implementation during post-heart surgery rehabilitation could improve the quality of the rehabilitation process and, in the end, the health of the patients. Although yoga and meditation are practiced by millions of people around the world and their positive effects have been recorded, the use of these approaches remains underestimated by the research community. As mentioned by Thabane and colleagues, the common idea behind how a pilot study is presented by multiple sources is the conduction of a study in advance of a larger, more comprehensive investigation [40]. They also suggested that feasibility should be a part of the pilot study. In accordance with this, the present pilot study was conducted in a way that meets CONSORT (Consolidated Standards of Reporting Trials) criteria ([41], Figure 1, Supplement Table S1). The objectives of this study were as follows: the investigation of the changes in retinal microvasculature in cardiac patients undergoing cardiac rehabilitation; the comparison of three different rehabilitation approaches (standard rehabilitation therapy, standard rehabilitation therapy plus meditation, and standard rehabilitation therapy plus yoga) in cardiac patients; and the examination of the possibility of capturing changes caused by cardiac rehabilitation using retinal imaging, which represents a novel and promising strategy in cardiovascular health evaluation [42–47]. We also aimed to provide preliminary data about the given topic and highlight the importance of this research gap to encourage further research.

This study hypothesizes that changes in retinal microvasculature will be observed in cardiac patients undergoing cardiac rehabilitation; there will be differences in outcomes among the three rehabilitation approaches; retinal imaging will be a reliable method for capturing changes over the study and evaluating cardiovascular health in a non-invasive manner; and this study will provide preliminary data with in order to address the importance of this research and contribute to future research endeavors.

2. Methods

This pilot, randomized, and single-blinded (investigator) clinical study was carried out from October to December 2019. Patients who had experienced coronary events were eligible for in-patient rehabilitation at the Rehabilitation Center of the Pensionsversicherungsanstalt in St. Radegund. The standard period of rehabilitation in St. Radegund is four weeks. In this study, the patients were randomly assigned to one of the three groups using a free, demo version of online software https://www.randomizer.at (accessed on 30 September 2019) for block randomization. This study was approved by the ethics committee and preregistered as a pilot clinical study at clinicaltrials.gov. The clinical study and data collection were performed in accordance with the Declaration of Helsinki (2013) of the World Medical Association. Every patient received detailed information about the study protocol and provided verbal and written informed consent. The flow of the study participants is shown in Figure 1.

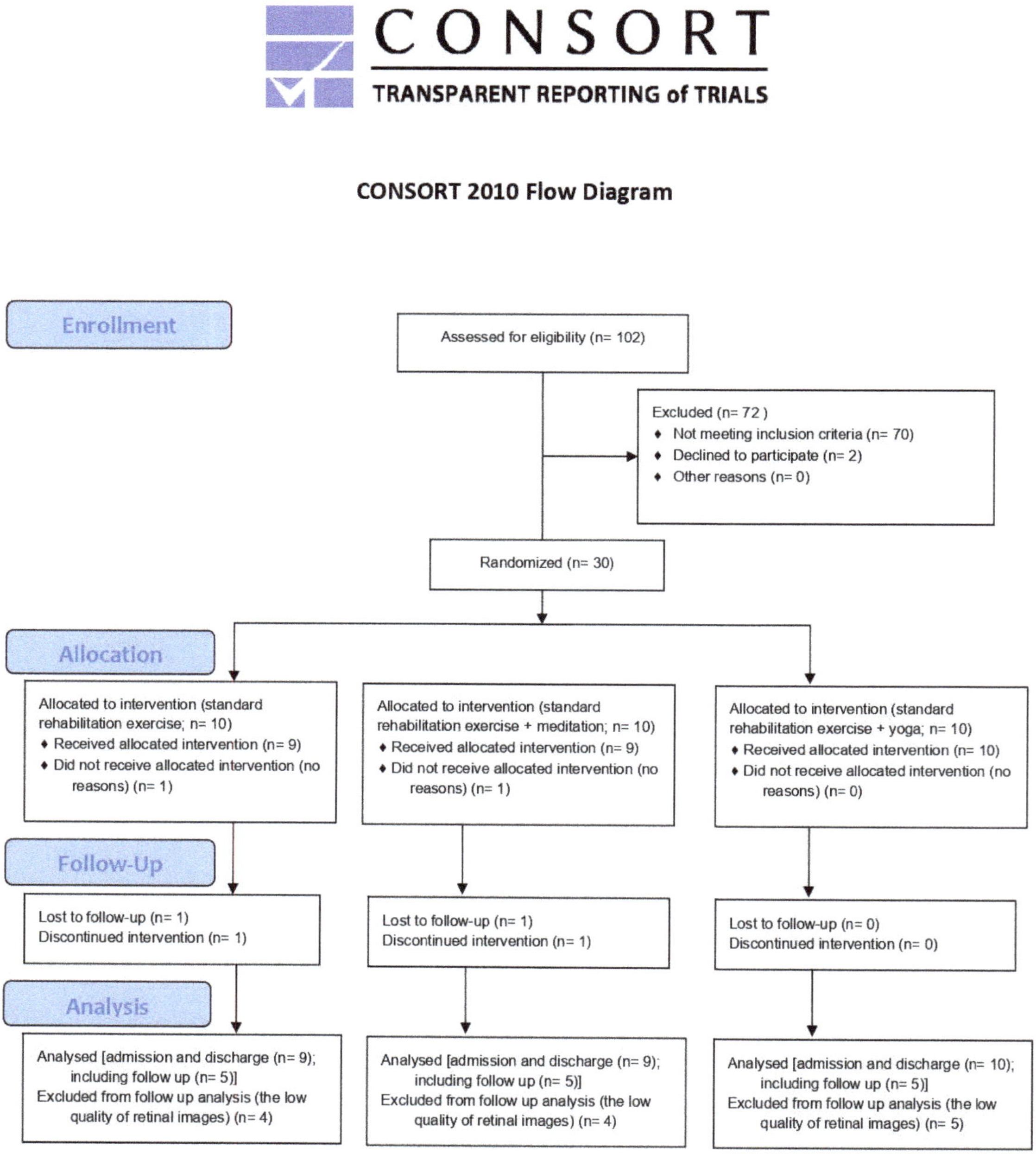

Figure 1. CONSORT flow diagram.

2.1. Participants

Over the duration of two weeks, patients who arrived at the clinic to start their 4-week rehabilitation program and who met the strict inclusion criteria were enrolled in this study (Figure 1). On the day of admission, all patients underwent a clinical examination (general medical history and clinical examination), including ECG. The medications which were taken by the patients in the study included cardiovascular agents (such as ACE inhibitors, beta blockers, calcium channel blockers, diuretics, and statins), analgesics (such as paracetamol, ibuprofen, and diclofenac), antiplatelet and anticoagulant agents (such as aspirin, clopidogrel, and warfarin), respiratory agents (such as bronchodilators and corticosteroids), and gastrointestinal agents (such as proton pump inhibitors, H2 blockers, and antacids).

This study employed a parallel-group randomized controlled trial design with an allocation ratio of 1:1:1. The thirty patients included were randomly assigned to three study groups—control, meditation, and yoga (Figure 2, Table 1). While the control group only received the standard rehabilitation exercise program, TM and yoga groups received, in addition to the standard rehabilitation therapy, either double the amount of meditation or yoga sessions of 20 min per day, respectively (Figure 2). The given groups performed meditation or yoga exercises according to a plan, as mentioned later and in the work of Rudlof and colleagues [21].

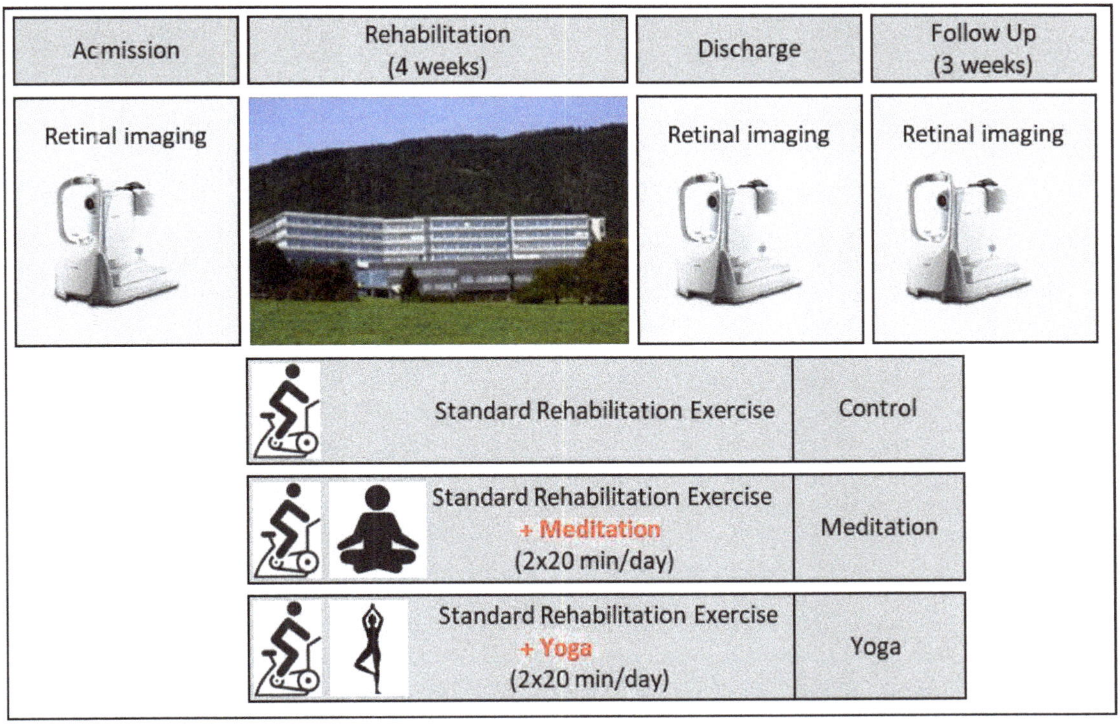

Figure 2. Overview of the study protocol (adapted from Rudlof and colleagues [21]).

Table 1. Characteristics of the study sample, excluding two dropouts from the beginning of the study. Data are shown as mean ± SD.

Characteristics	Control	Meditation	Yoga	Total Sample
Male (n)	8 (89%)	8 (89%)	6 (60%)	22 (79%)
Female (n)	1 (11%)	1 (11%)	4 (40%)	6 (21%)
Age (years)	59.33 (±7.81)	59.56 (±7.84)	59.20 (±12.09)	59.36 (±9.22)
Height (cm)	176.72 (±7.11)	173.44 (±7.73)	170.20 (±8.79)	173.34 (±8.12)
Weight (kg)	94.73 (±9.95)	79.56 (±19.22)	80.00 (±25.00)	84.59 (±20.23)
BMI (kg/m^2)	30.42 (±4.24)	26.31 (±5.10)	27.30 (±6.74)	27.99 (±5.59)

2.2. Sample Size

As there were no other studies we were aware of that investigated the effect of TM and/or yoga in the setting of cardiac rehabilitation, we conducted a pilot study with 30 participants (10 in each group). The primary outcomes measured included changes in endothelial function, which were assessed through various modalities such as flow-mediated dilatation, pulse wave velocity, retinal imaging, and cardiopostural interactions.

2.3. Eligibility Criteria

Participants had to meet the following criteria to be included in this study. They needed to be recovering from one of these conditions: myocardial infarction, ST-elevation myocardial infarction, non-ST-elevation myocardial infarction, acute coronary syndrome, coronary artery disease with percutaneous coronary intervention, or a coronary artery bypass graft. The inclusion age was from 40 to 80 years, and participants had to be inpatient admissions at the Cardiac Rehabilitation Center St. Radegund. The exclusion criteria were as follows: patients who had to be monitored because of severe disease; patients with NYHA III or more; patients with a mini-mental score of less than 26; patients who were not sufficiently mobilized; and patients who regularly perform any kind of meditation techniques. No study participants suffered from retinopathies or eye problems.

2.4. Standard Rehabilitation Exercise Therapy

During the 4 weeks of cardiac rehabilitation, the patients received an individual therapy plan. The individual rehabilitation schedule was created for each patient according to the results of health check tests and their fitness level/condition/performance. The individual performance was assessed via cyclic ergometry. The rehabilitation program was multidisciplinary, containing an exercise part, physiotherapeutic treatment, nutrition support, psychological assistance, and rehabilitation nursing. The following exercises were available for the patients: bicycle or treadmill (with ECG monitoring); Nordic walking, hiking (in groups); gymnastics; strength, endurance, and mobility workouts; weightlifting under physiotherapeutic control; and swimming. All therapeutic units had a duration of 25 or 50 min. The exercise modality followed a standardized procedure. In general, the patients underwent 2400 min of standard rehabilitation exercise therapy in 4 weeks. All diagnostic and therapeutic processes were performed following the latest guidelines of the European Society of Cardiology (ESC).

The physiotherapeutic individual treatment included, for example, massages, lymphatic drainages, electro-therapy, etc. Nutritional support included education about mixed healthy diets provided by dieticians, including various educational seminars (such as lectures concerning cardiovascular risk factors). Psychological assistance, employing stress-reducing methods, was free to access for all patients depending on their individual needs. Additionally, relaxation sessions that patients could attend comprised progressive muscle relaxation, autogenic training, acupuncture massage, and dry water massage. The relaxation schedule was individually adapted depending on the patient's condition and preferences.

The staff members were trained for this special group of patients. Medical doctors, mainly specialists in internal medicine/cardiology or general practitioners, therapeutic staff, psychologists, dietologists, and nurses gave support in multiple aspects of patients' lives. The object of the therapeutic and diagnostic procedures is the restoration and strengthening of workability and participation in everyday life.

2.5. Standard Rehabilitation Exercise Therapy + Transcendental Meditation

In the beginning, before the study started, the patients received four introductory transcendental meditation lectures in which the method was learned via practice. Two TM professionals of the "Austrian Society of Maharishi Vedic Sciences" (Österreichische Gesellschaft für Maharishi Vedische Wissenschaft) held these introductory transcendental meditation lectures in which the participants learned the technique. Each of these first four introductory sessions lasted for about 1–1.5 h and took place on 4 consecutive days. To correctly learn the method, it was necessary to complete all four sessions in a row.

After the introductory lectures, the TM technique was practiced twice a day for 20 min, with one session in the morning (6:30–6:50) and one in the evening (16:30–16:50). Two group meetings per week and one individual personal meeting with the TM teacher (this allowed the patients to ask questions) guaranteed the right performance of TM by the patients.

2.6. Standard Rehabilitation Exercise Therapy + Yoga

In the beginning, before the study started, the patients in this group received a 20 min workshop where they learned how to perform yoga exercises. The yoga workshop was held by a yoga expert.

Afterward, yoga sessions were included in the regular/standard exercise. The yoga group performed yoga, which included physical poses (Asanas), body scan, breathing exercises (Pranayamas), and affirmations, at the same time slots as those described for the TM group. It was practiced twice a day for 20 min, with one session in the morning (6:30–6:50) and one in the evening (16:30–16:50).

2.7. Study Protocol

Patients were tested at three separate time points: the first measurement (admission/baseline measurement) was taken one day after admission and before any kind of rehabilitation, the second measurement was taken four weeks later (discharge measurement) at the end of the rehabilitation program, and the third measurement (follow up measurement) was conducted three weeks after discharge (Figure 2). The measurements were performed within one day of each other at fixed times (9:00, 10:30, 13:00, 14:30, and 16:00) and were individually repeated at the same time (admission, discharge, and follow-up interventions/control). While the current study involves the same number of participants as the large comprehensive project, it serves as a pilot study in terms of measurement comprehensiveness. The present pilot study focused solely on the retinal microcirculation approach, providing a unique perspective within the broader scope of the main project. The whole project encompasses a broader range of measurements, for example, tension myography [48] and cardiovascular parameter evaluation using the Task Force Monitor® (CNSystems, Graz, Austria) [21]. The detailed protocol is shown in the previous research [21].

2.8. Retinal Assessment

The retinal images (resolution of 1536 × 1536) focused on the optic disc of the right eye were collected at 3 points according to the study protocol. They were taken by a trained person using a non-mydriatic digital retinal camera, Canon CR-2 (Canon Medical Systems Europe B.V., Amstelveen, The Netherlands). This was followed by the allocation, organization, and preparation of retinal images for analysis. The analysis was performed by a trained grader blinded from any previous knowledge about the details of the study using the semi-automated software (version 2.1.1) MONA Reva (VITO, Boeretang, Mol, Belgium). The diameters of retinal microvessels in an area 0.5 to 1 the size of the optic disc radius, determined from the optic disc margin, were automatically analyzed. Subsequently, the trained grader checked, corrected, and labeled vessels (arterioles, venules). The Knudson formula was used to calculate retinal parameters ((central retinal artery equivalent (CRAE), central retinal vein equivalent (CRVE) and artery-to-vein ratio (AVR)) from the 6 largest retinal arterioles and the 6 largest retinal venules [49–55]. An example of the fundus image taken during the study is displayed in Figure 3.

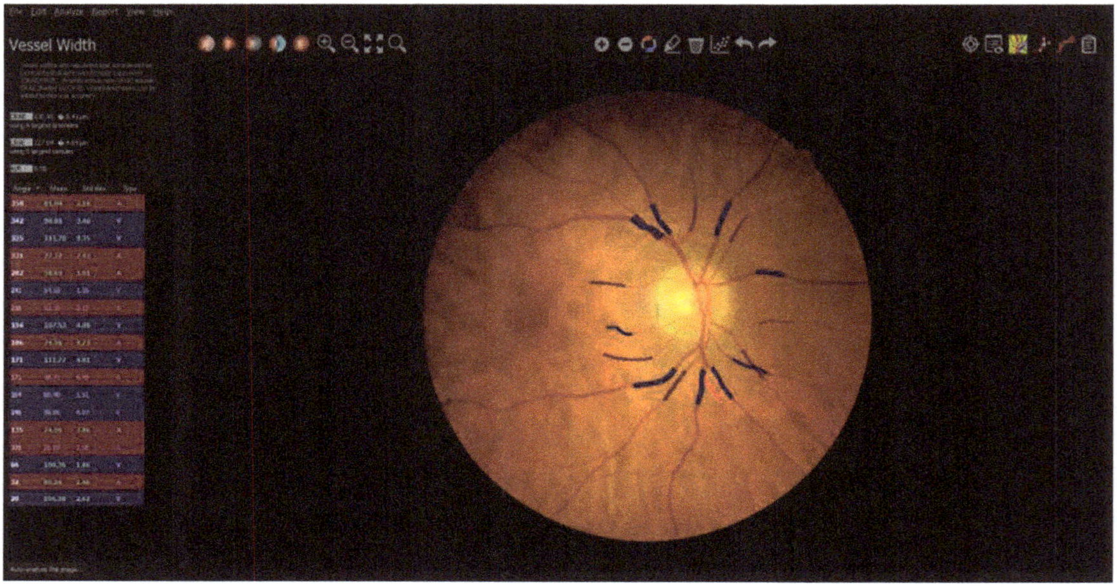

Figure 3. An optic disc focused image of the retina displayed in software (version 2.1.1) MONA-REVA during the analysis process. The table on the left side of the picture shows the list of the analyzed vessels. Arteries are displayed in red and venules are shown in blue. Boldly displayed vessels in the table, which correspond to the six biggest arteries and six largest venules from the picture, were used for the calculation of CRAE and CRVE. Central retinal artery equivalent (CRAE); central retinal vein equivalent (CRVE).

2.9. Statistical Analysis

All retinal data were checked to determine the normality of the distribution via the Shapiro–Wilk test. For the comparison of retinal parameters at the three different time points, repeated measures ANOVA was performed, using the rehabilitation type as the between-subject factor. Statistical significance was determined in relation to a two-tailed p-value of $p < 0.05$. Data were analyzed using IBM SPSS Version 28.0 (IBM Corp., Armonk, NY, USA). Continuous variables are expressed as mean ± standard deviation (SD).

3. Results

Overall, 30 patients (24 males, 6 females; mean age: 59.36 (±9.22); height: 173.34 (±8.12); weight: 84.59 (±20.23); and BMI: 27.99 (±5.59)) were recruited in this pilot, randomized clinical study (Table 1). In total, 2 patients dropped out at the beginning of the study (without further explanation), and 13 additional dropouts (caused by low quality of retinal images) were noticed during follow-up measurements. Therefore, the follow-up measurements could be only performed with 50% of the patients (5 in each group). Table 1 summarizes the basic characteristics of the study participants.

Retinal Microvasculature

Table 2 summarizes the analyzed retinal parameters of the three groups.

Considering CRAE, the repeated measures ANOVA revealed neither a main effect for time point (admission, discharge, follow-up: F(2,24) = 0.890, p = 0.424) nor a group effect (F(2,12) = 1.236, p = 0.325), and the interaction was also non-significant (F(4,24) = 0.600, p = 0.666). Similarly, we found no main effect for the time point (F(2,22) = 0.483, p = 0.620), group (F(2,11) = 0.500, p = 0.620) or the interaction (F(4,22) = 1.477, p = 0.243) for CRVE. Also, the analysis of the AV ratio did not show statistical significance for any effect (time point: F(2,22) = 1.821, p = 0.185; group: F(2,11) = 0.788, p = 0.479; interaction: F(4,22) = 1.316, p = 0.295). Overall, we saw no significant effect for intervention, and thus rehabilitation, or between patients' groups with regard to retinal microcirculation parameters.

Due to the large drop out of patients in the follow-up measurements, we also only compared the time points—admission and discharge—that were available for 28 patients. However, the statistical analyses correspondingly showed no significant differences between the three groups (Table 3).

Table 2. The effect of meditation or yoga in addition to a standard rehabilitation exercise program on retinal arteriolar and venular diameters in patients after heart surgery. Data are shown as mean ± SD (control, meditation, Yoga) at the respective timepoints (admission, discharge, follow-up). N—number of patients in each group; Medit.—meditation; CRAE—central retinal artery equivalent; CRVE—central retinal vein equivalent; AVR—artery-to-vein ratio.

Parameter	Group	Admission	Discharge	Follow-Up	N	*p*-Value
CRAE (μm)	Control	131.30 ± 13.20	132.03 ± 16.48	133.75 ± 14.32	5	0.666
	Medit.	140.23 ± 8.74	139.11 ± 7.88	140.20 ± 8.86	5	
	Yoga	146.98 ± 14.66	142.75 ± 16.99	145.00 ± 12.02	5	
CRVE (μm)	Control	211.67 ± 12.30	205.21 ± 7.07	204.62 ± 5.40	5	0.243
	Medit.	213.70 ± 23.27	215.30 ± 20.30	217.01 ± 19.61	5	
	Yoga	210.49 ± 9.21	219.51 ± 17.11	215.56 ± 19.17	5	
AVR	Control	0.63 ± 0.08	0.63 ± 0.07	0.63 ± 0.07	5	0.295
	Medit.	0.67 ± 0.04	0.66 ± 0.04	0.66 ±0.01	5	
	Yoga	0.70 ± 0.05	0.65 ± 0.04	0.65 ± 0.05	5	

Table 3. The effect of meditation or yoga in addition to a standard rehabilitation exercise program on retinal arteriolar and venular diameters in patients after heart surgery. Data show group ± SDs (Control, Meditation, Yoga) at the respective timepoints (Admission, Discharge). Data are shown as mean ± SD. N—number of patients in each group; Medit.—Meditation; CRAE—central retinal artery equivalent; CRVE—central retinal vein equivalent; AVR—artery-to-vein ratio.

Parameter	Group	Admission	Discharge	N	*p*-Value
CRAE (μm)	Control	141.4 ± 15.78	141.91 ± 17.65	9	0.936
	Medit.	135.84 ± 12.23	135.84 ± 9.35	9	
	Yoga	138.56 ± 13.06	138.16 ± 11.38	10	
CRVE (μm)	Control	212.28 ± 8.41	215.56 ± 11.13	9	0.193
	Medit.	208.55 ± 24.45	212.23 ± 20.84	9	
	Yoga	212.82 ± 14.09	214.31 ± 13.98	10	
AVR	Control	0.67 ± 0.08	0.66 ± 0.06	9	0.181
	Medit.	0.66 ± 0.07	0.64 ± 0.06	9	
	Yoga	0.65 ± 0.06	0.65 ± 0.05	10	

For CRAE measurements, there were no significant effects for time point (pre-post: F(1,25) = 0.001, p = 0.970), group (F(2,25) = 0.439, p = 0.649), or their interaction (F(2,25) = 0.066, p = 0.936). Similarly, and also for the CRVE measurements, no significant changes were observed between admission and discharge (F(1,25) = 1.794, p = 0.193), group (F(2,25) = 0.146, p = 0.865), or their interaction (F(2,25) = 0.106, p = 0.900). Also, the AV ratio showed that the factors included had no effect (admission–discharge: F(1,25) = 1.891, p = 0.181; group: F(2,25) = 0.143, p = 0.867; interaction: F(2,25) = 0.028, p = 0.972).

4. Discussion

We did not find any differences in retinal microcirculation parameters over time between the three rehabilitation groups: those receiving standard rehabilitation exercise program only, those practicing yoga, and those practicing TM. Nonetheless, our results are novel and encourage future research as there is an evident lack of peer-reviewed articles from the Western world covering topics of meditation and yoga and no previous study has examined cardiovascular health via retinal imaging—a promising, non-invasive, and cost-effective technique [42]—in cardiac patients during cardiac rehabilitation.

The positive effects of exercise on cardiovascular health are very well known [56–61]. The acute effects of exercise are manifested via the elevation in cardiac stroke volume and HR, an increase in cardiac output, which coupled with a transient increase in systemic vascular resistance, increases mean arterial BP. However, it was confirmed by numerous quantitative studies that long-term exercise not only promotes a reduction in HR and BP at rest but also has an impact on a lot of other parameters related to cardiovascular health. Moreover, different types of exercise approaches are important therapeutic treatments for patients with cardiovascular diseases and help in rehabilitation after cardiac surgeries. Hambrecht and colleagues investigated the effect of exercise on coronary endothelial function in 19 CAD patients randomized to either an exercise-training group (10 patients) or a control group (9 patients) [58]. After 4 weeks of study, increased response to acetylcholine and a 29% increase in coronary blood-flow reserve were observed in the exercise-training group, which showed improvement in endothelium-dependent vasodilatation. A meta-analysis from Fagard showed that dynamic physical training, performed 3–5 times (30–60 min/session) per week, decreases BP by an average of 3.4/2.4 mmHg [59]. A systematic review and meta-analysis of 48 trials (6 or more months of follow-up) with 8940 patients concluded that, compared with usual care, exercise-based cardiac rehabilitation is associated with reduced all-cause mortality, better improvement in lipid profile, a reduction in systolic BP (SBP), and lower rates of self-reported smoking [60]. Another meta-analysis involved 72 trials, 105 study groups, and 3936 participants and investigated the effects of endurance training on BP [61]. It was found that training reduces resting and daytime ambulatory BP by 3.0/2.4 mm Hg and 3.3/3.5 mm Hg, respectively. Moreover, the reduction in resting BP was even higher in the hypertensive study groups ($-6.9/-4.9$ mm Hg). Other results were seen in the reduction in systemic vascular resistance by 7.1%, plasma norepinephrine by 29%, and plasma renin activity by 20%. Body weight dropped by 1.2 kg, waist circumference fell by 2.8 cm, percent body fat fell by 1.4%, and the homeostasis model assessment index of insulin resistance fell by 0.31 IU/L^{-1}. Additionally, HDL increased by 0.032 $mmol/L^{-1}$. With regard to these results mentioned above, the effects of aerobic endurance training on cardiovascular health, via a favorable impact on cardiovascular risk factors, are evident. It is possible that similar effects were seen in our study cohorts, as all three groups that we studied received similar but rigorous standard exercise therapy. However, we did not observe any significant changes in retinal microcirculation parameters, not even between three different time points. Moreover, the retinal imaging technique is a sensitive approach, especially when it comes to sample size. On the other hand, individualized and non-uniform exercise training, which has a lot of different exercise options to choose from, could be also an important factor that limits the capture of significant results.

In a systematic review and meta-analysis, Chu and colleagues looked at the effectiveness of yoga in modifying risk factors for cardiovascular disease, and a no-exercise group and an exercise group were used as controls [22]. When they compared the yoga group with non-exercise controls, the yoga group showed significant improvement in BMI (-0.77 kg/m^2), SBP (-5.21 mmHg), LDL (-12.14 mg/dL), and HDL (3.20 mg/dL), as well as in body weight (−2.32 kg), diastolic BP (DBP) (−4.98 mmHg), total cholesterol (−18.48 mg/dL), triglycerides (−25.89 mg/dL), and HR (−5.27 beats/min). However, there was no significant difference between the yoga and exercise approaches. Therefore, yoga seemed to be a comparably effective treatment for improving cardiovascular profile via exercise. Also, Murugesan and colleagues reported that yoga has a positive effect on the cardiovascular system and is effective in the treatment of hypertension [62]. Thirty-three hypertensives (35–65 years) participated in a clinical trial and were assigned to three groups (1. yoga exercise, 2. medical treatment, 3. neither yoga nor medical treatment). The yoga group performed yoga exercises for one hour in the morning and in the evening, and the medical treatment group took one drug every day for 11 weeks. The capability to control hypertension was investigated for both groups. Both treatments, yoga as well as medications, were effective in controlling hypertension as the study participants showed significant decreases in SBP, DBP, pulse rate, and body weight. Our study participants took part in yoga exercises twice a day for 20 min over the course of 4 weeks. It is possible that the shorter daily time of yoga practice as well as the total duration of the study, only 4 weeks compared to 11 weeks in the study mentioned above, prevented us from seeing any significant effects in the parameters of retinal microcirculation. Moreover, even though yoga has an impact on psychological well-being, stress reduction, and overall quality of life, we did not measure those aspects. This could, potentially pose confounders or variables that were not controlled for in the study. Unaccounted psychological factors, subjective well-being, and heterogeneity in participant responses to yoga may also partially explain our non-significant results.

A systematic review and meta-analysis investigating the impact of yoga on cardiovascular disease risk factors showed the beneficial effects of yoga ($p < 0.05$) on SBP (reduced by 5.85 mm Hg), DBP (reduced by 4.12 mm Hg), HR (reduced by 6.59 beats/min), respiratory rate (reduced by 0.93 breaths/min), abdominal obesity (decrease in waist/hip ratio and waist circumference), lipid profile (decrease in LDL, total cholesterol, triglycerides and increase in HDL), hemoglobin A1c (reduced by 0.45%),O and insulin resistance (reduced by 0.19) relative to usual care or no intervention [23]. Pal and colleagues investigated the effect of yoga practice on cardiovascular health in patients with coronary artery disease [63]. Overall, 170 patients were assigned to either a yoga group [35–40 min/day, five days/week) or a non-yoga group for six months. They also noted significant reductions in BMI, SBP, DBP, HR, total cholesterol, triglycerides, and LDL in the yoga group. Therefore, yoga may be a helpful intervention for patients with coronary artery disease. Despite an identical number of yoga sessions, the total duration of the study was six months, and was hence six times longer than the present study. This may be the reason we did not achieve significant changes in the variables we investigated.

Another study included 130 patients with heart failure and assigned them to a yoga group (standard medical therapy + yoga (60 min/day, three days/week, a total of 36 sessions)) or a control group (standard medical therapy) [27]. They observed a significant reduction in HR and BP in the yoga group compared to the control group. Moreover, the reduction in LF and LF-HF ratio and elevation in HF in the yoga group showed improved parasympathetic activity and decreased sympathetic activity. Although this study took 12 weeks, the overall duration of the yoga exercises during the whole study was similar to ours. Compared to the present study, yoga exercises were more intense for our patients; therefore, we would expect to see significant changes. However, while their study included 130 participants, our pilot study had only 30, with additional dropouts recorded during the protocol. Those and the already abovementioned reasons may be behind our non-significant results.

A case-control study included 100 subjects (50 controls (not doing any type of physical exercise), and 50 study subjects (practicing yoga for 5 years)) above 40 years of age [64]. They found that the study group had significantly lower SBP and DBP. Five years and one month is a very big difference in study duration, and this is probably the reason why similar results were not reflected in our measurements. Slower breathing rate is a typical part of yoga exercises. A total of 79 mild hypertensive individuals with BP > 140/90 mm Hg were enrolled in a study and assigned to either the treatment or control group [65]. Patients in the treatment group performed a 15 min/day session of device-guided breathing exercises. We obtained BP and HR results, self-measured at home every morning throughout the 10-week, from both groups. Device-guided breathing exercises caused a reduction in SPB and DBP (5.5/3.6 mm Hg at the clinic and 5.4/3.2 mm Hg at home). Although this study did not deal directly with yoga exercises, the slower breathing rate is a typical part of yoga exercises. The daily duration was shorter, but the study lasted 2.5 times longer compared to the present study. Perhaps a longer period of time with shorter daily duration of breathing exercises, compared to a shorter intervention period and more intense exposure to yoga, has a more beneficial effect.

The beneficial effects of TM have previously been published [66]. Dillbeck and Orme-Johnson observed acute reductions in respiratory rate and plasma lactate in the TM group compared to the control group, which was characterized by increased basal skin resistance. Moreover, we observed lower baseline HR, respiratory rate, plasma lactate level, and spontaneous skin resistance responses outside of meditation in the TM group. Mindfulness-based stress reduction (MBSR) is an eight-week program offering intensive mindfulness training to assist people with stress, anxiety, or depression. Fifty-six patients with unmedicated prehypertension were randomly assigned to MBSR or progressive muscle relaxation (PMR) groups [17]. The study lasted for 8 weeks, with treatment sessions of 2.5 h each week. The MBSR group showed a 4.8 mm Hg and 1.9 mm Hg reductions in SBP and DBP, respectively, compared to a 0.7 mm Hg reduction in SBP and 1.2 mm Hg increase in DBP in the PMR group. The total duration of meditation during the study was comparable to the present study, but our study lasted half as long (4 weeks vs. 8 weeks) and the exposure to meditation was therefore less intense. Similar to what we saw with yoga, perhaps a longer and less intensive form of therapy may have a greater effect. Moreover, similarly, as was mentioned in the discussion of yoga, the absence of measurements related to psychological well-being, stress reduction, and overall quality of life in the study may potentially present confounding issues that were not controlled for in the analysis of retinal microcirculation.

A single-blind study with a 3 month follow-up investigated the effect of 3 different approaches (TM, PMR, or lifestyle modification exercise) on the treatment of mild hypertension in 127 elderly African Americans (aged 55 to 85 years) [67]. It was observed that both TM and PMR reduced SBP (10.7 mmHg and 4.7 mmHg) and DBP (6.4 mmHg, 3.3 mmHg). However, the TM approach was approximately twice as effective when the reductions in the TM group were significantly greater than those seen in the PMR group. As in present study, the subjects conducted TM twice daily (morning and evening) for 20 min per session. The differences lie in the length of the Schneider study (3 months [67] vs. our intervention duration of only 4 weeks). This, along with multiple reasons already mentioned, could have contributed to the lack of changes in retinal microcirculation parameters in our patient population.

A meta-analysis from 2008 including normotensive, prehypertensive, and hypertensive individuals (ages from adolescent to senior) compared BP changes in TM and the control group [25]. Average reductions of 4.7 mmHg in SBP and 3.2 mmHg in DBP in TM groups were observed when compared with control groups. Additionally, subgroup analyses of hypertensive groups and high-quality studies showed similar BP values. Another meta-analysis performed by Rainforth and colleagues investigated the effects of stress reduction programs (biofeedback, relaxation-assisted biofeedback, progressive muscle relaxation, stress management training, and TM program] on changes in BP [68]. To sum up, only TM showed a significant reduction in SBP (5 mmHg, $p = 0.002$) and DBP (2.8 mmHg, $p = 0.02$). Two additional studies showed that TM also has beneficial effects on insulin resistance and lipid profiles. One of the studies lasted for 16 weeks, with 103 participants with coronary heart disease (CHD), and was randomized to either TM or a health education (HE) group to examine the efficacy of TM on components of metabolic syndrome and CHD [18]. The TM group had two introductory lectures (1.5 h each), personal interview (10–15 min), personal instruction (1–1.5 h), 3 group meetings (1.5 h each), and follow-up and maintenance meetings (1.5 h) twice per week during the first 4 weeks and then weekly. The HE group had the same number, length, and frequency of group meetings with health educators. The TM group showed favorable changes in SBP ($p = 0.04$), insulin resistance ($p = 0.01$), and HRV (HF; $p = 0.07$) compared with the control group. The increasing HF values suggests that there is autonomic regulation, particular increased parasympathetic activity, involved in the mechanism of TM's effect on cardiovascular health. Additionally, a small study where Cooper and Aygen compared 12 patients with hypercholesterolemia regularly practicing TM (20 min/day, 13 months) with 11 control subjects displayed a 10% ($p < 0.005$) reduction in fasting serum cholesterol levels in the TM group compared with the control group [24]. The first of these two studies again had a longer duration, as well as less frequent sessions and a bigger sample size, than our own. All these factors could have contributed to the differences from the findings in our study. The second study was like the present study only with a small sample size. However, they had shorter meditation sessions per day (20 min vs. 2 × 20 min in present study). However, the overall duration of the respective study's meditation therapy was 13 months, which is a big difference compared to our 4-week intervention. It cannot be forgotten that the retinal imaging technique is a sensitive approach, especially when it comes to sample size, and together with the mentioned confounders and other reasons may contribute to the non-significant results of the present study.

Previous studies have also shown the effect of these two alternative approaches on HRV and the autonomic nervous system. Yoga, as well as TM, showed a boost in parasympathetic activity and the silencing of sympathetic activity, which is considered the main their mechanism of action affecting the cardiovascular system [12,24–27]. We did not, however, measure autonomic function via heart rate variability.

5. Summary

To summarize the results of the present study, we did not observe significant changes in retinal microvasculature as an effect of three different cardiac rehabilitation approaches, neither between rehabilitation groups nor between different measurement time points. Previous research proved that exercise has a favorable impact on cardiovascular risk factors. It improves the ability of the mitochondrion to adjust cardiac metabolism, causes a reduction in oxidative stress, and increases the cardiac reserve capacity. Based on the previous research, we hypothesized that four weeks of cardiac rehabilitation program would be enough to transform cardiovascular changes into changes in retinal microvasculature. Moreover, we compared the standard exercise rehabilitation approach with either yoga or TM, and also compared these approaches with each other. Similarly, as an exercise, the positive effects of meditation and yoga on mental as well as cardiovascular health are known [9–12,19–21]. We believed that four weeks of yoga or meditation in addition to standard rehabilitation would be strong enough to surpass the effect of standard exercise rehabilitation itself. We expected these cardiovascular changes to be transformed into changes in retinal microvasculature. This novel approach to measuring the physiological effects in cardiac patients undergoing cardiac rehabilitation and retinal imaging presents a promising, non-invasive, and cost-effective technique for cardiovascular health evaluation [28–37].

We believe that the small sample size, with additional dropouts in follow-up measurements as well as differences in the duration of sessions and overall interventions, could have masked the significant results that were expected. According to the previous research, it was observed that perhaps a longer and less intensive therapy may have a greater effect. Furthermore, individualized and non-uniform exercise training, with a lot of different exercise options to choose, from could be also an important factor that limits the capture of significant results. In addition, even though yoga and meditation have an impact on psychological well-being, stress reduction, and the overall quality of life, we did not measure these factors, and they can potentially present confounders or variables that were not controlled for in the study. The psychological factors unaccounted for, subjective well-being, and heterogeneity in participant responses to yoga and meditation may also partially explain our non-significant results. Finally, the retinal imaging technique is a sensitive approach, especially when it comes to sample size, and may contribute to difficulties with observing the significances within the present study.

6. Limitations

One of the limitations of the study is that we did not include a large number of patients. We believe that the small sample size could have masked significant results when three measurement time points were used, with only five patients per group. However, we do not think this is a problem, as the present study was a pilot study that aimed to assess microvascular changes. The obtained data will provide us with information (such as determining how possible the design of a study is in reality or allowing us to calculate sample sizes) for larger epidemiological studies. The medications that have been taken by the participants could be considered as a limitation that could affect the results of the study; however, cardiac patients typically take these types of medications. The present study groups were balanced in terms medication usage, keeping the quality of our study groups stable, and we do not believe that the medications taken by the patients in the present study affected the results of the study. Moreover, in this repeat measurement study, the same patients were assessed pre- and post-intervention. Another limitation of the present clinical study is that we could not carry out the follow-up in all the patients. This was largely because the COVID-19 pandemic occurred during that period, which limited our access to patients, and hence we experienced a lot of missing data. A potential limitation of our study is also that the interventions (yoga and TM) were only applied for a brief period. A comparison of the present study results with other studies indicates that a longer and less intensive therapy (yoga/TM) could have a greater beneficial effect on retinal microvasculature than a shorter and more intensive approach. In addition, even though yoga and meditation have an impact on psychological well-being, stress reduction, and overall quality of life, we did not measure those aspects, and these factors can potentially present confounders or variables that were not controlled for in the study. Furthermore, individualized and non-uniform exercise training, with a lot of different exercise options to choose, from could be also an important factor and limit the capture of significant results. Lastly, the high sensitivity of the retinal imaging technique, especially when it comes to sample size, could also pose a limitation of this study as the method may not be able to capture differences in given parameters. However, we do not believe this was the case as all pictures were captured and analyzed by trained personnel of the Medical University of Graz.

Despite the above limitations, the present clinical study provides novelties in terms of rehabilitation approaches after cardiac surgery. In addition to the exercise protocols that are widely used during cardiac rehabilitation, non-pharmacological approaches, such as yoga and meditation, can also be incorporated. Furthermore, the present study presents novel results, as there is a lack of research in this area, and shows that cardiovascular health can be routinely assessed non-invasively by the retinal imaging approach. The combination of these underestimated rehabilitation approaches and the assessment by retinal imaging, which presents novelty and a promising approach in cardiovascular health evaluation, ensures the significance of the present pilot study. As our results were not conclusive, we suggest that future research should include longer periods of breathing exercises and yoga to examine the potential effects of yoga and TM on retinal microcirculation and overall cardiovascular health.

7. Conclusions

The present pilot study introduced complementary rehabilitation approaches, including yoga and meditation, for cardiac surgery patients, and explored the use of retinal imaging as a non-invasive method to evaluate cardiovascular health. Although no significant changes in retinal microcirculation were observed, the findings provide foundational insights for future studies examining the integration of health promotion practices such as yoga and meditation into cardiac rehabilitation. The study also highlights the need for more comprehensive research in this area, particularly from Western populations, and underscores the potential of retinal imaging techniques in assessing cardiovascular health. Furthermore, we encourage the research community to conduct larger-scale studies to validate these approaches. Studies should utilize longer intervention durations and more robust methodologies in order to better understand the physiological impacts of yoga and meditation on retinal vascular health.

Author Contributions: Conceptualization, P.M., A.D., R.P. and N.G.; methodology, A.S., K.S.-Z., B.S., R.P. and N.G.; validation, N.G.; formal analysis, A.S. and K.S.-Z.; data curation, A.S., K.S.-Z., B.S., M.E.R. and T.O.B.; investigation A.S., K.S.-Z., B.S., M.E.R. and T.O.B.; writing—original draft preparation, A.S.; writing—review and editing, K.S.-Z., B.S., M.E.R., P.M., A.D., P.M.F., B.N.N.-C. and N.G. All authors have read and agreed to the published version of the manuscript.

Funding: This research received no external funding.

Institutional Review Board Statement: The ethics approval proposition was admitted on 7 June 2019 by the Ethics Committee of the Medical University of Graz (EK 31-443 ex 18/19) and approved on 16 July 2019. The study was preregistered as a pilot clinical study (Nr. NCT05035758; TMY_Rehab) and submitted on 19 August 2021 at clinicaltrials.gov. The clinical study and data collection were performed in accordance with the Declaration of Helsinki (2013) of the WMA (the World Medical Association). Every patient received detailed information about the study protocol and provided verbal and written informed consent.

Informed Consent Statement: Written informed consent was obtained from all subjects involved in the study.

Data Availability Statement: All data generated or analyzed during this study are included in this published article. For any specific additional inquiries or requests for further information, please contact the corresponding author of this manuscript.

Acknowledgments: We are grateful to all patients who attended this study as well as to all staff of the Cardiac Rehabilitation Clinic in St. Radegund, a facility of the Austrian retirement insurance PVA (Pensionsversicherungsanstalt) who helped with running this study.

Conflicts of Interest: The authors declare no conflict of interest.

References

1. Roth, G.A.; Mensah, G.A.; Johnson, C.O.; Addolorato, G.; Ammirati, E.; Baddour, L.M.; Barengo, N.C.; Beaton, A.Z.; Benjamin, E.J.; Benziger, C.P.; et al. Global Burden of Cardiovascular Diseases and Risk Factors, 1990–2019: Update From the GBD 2019 Study. *J. Am. Coll. Cardiol.* **2020**, *76*, 2982–3021. [CrossRef] [PubMed]
2. Heart Surgery-What Is Heart Surgery? | NHLBI, NIH. Available online: https://www.nhlbi.nih.gov/health/heart-surgery (accessed on 21 December 2023).
3. Rippe, J.M. Lifestyle Strategies for Risk Factor Reduction, Prevention, and Treatment of Cardiovascular Disease. *Am. J. Lifestyle Med.* **2018**, *13*, 204–212. [CrossRef] [PubMed]
4. Dibben, G.O.; Faulkner, J.; Oldridge, N.; Rees, K.; Thompson, D.R.; Zwisler, A.-D.; Taylor, R.S. 6 Exercise-based cardiac rehabilitation for coronary heart disease—An updated cochrane systematic review and meta-analysis. *Heart* **2022**, *108*, A4.
5. Schneider, R.H.; Alexander, C.N.; Staggers, F.; Rainforth, M.; Salerno, J.W.; Hartz, A.; Arndt, S.; Barnes, V.A.; Nidich, S.I. Long-Term Effects of Stress Reduction on Mortality in Persons $\geq$55 Years of Age With Systemic Hypertension. *Am. J. Cardiol.* **2005**, *95*, 1060–1064. [CrossRef]
6. Osborne, M.T.; Shin, L.M.; Mehta, N.N.; Pitman, R.K.; Fayad, Z.A.; Tawakol, A. Disentangling the Links Between Psychosocial Stress and Cardiovascular Disease. *Circ. Cardiovasc. Imaging* **2020**, *13*, e010931. [CrossRef]
7. Dar, T.; Radfar, A.; Abohashem, S.; Pitman, R.K.; Tawakol, A.; Osborne, M.T. Psychosocial Stress and Cardiovascular Disease. *Curr. Treat. Options Cardiovasc. Med.* **2019**, *21*, 1–17. [CrossRef]
8. International Yoga Day: Discover the Power of Yoga–CircleDNA. Available online: https://circledna.com/blog/international-yoga-day-discover-the-power-of-yoga/ (accessed on 14 November 2024).
9. Guddeti, R.R.; Dang, G.; Williams, M.A.; Alla, V.M. Role of Yoga in Cardiac Disease and Rehabilitation. *J. Cardiopulm. Rehabil. Prev.* **2019**, *39*, 146–152. [CrossRef]
10. Manchanda, S.C.; Madan, K. Yoga and meditation in cardiovascular disease. *Clin. Res. Cardiol.* **2014**, *103*, 675–680. [CrossRef]
11. Woodyard, C. Exploring the therapeutic effects of yoga and its ability to increase quality of life. *Int. J. Yoga* **2011**, *4*, 49–54. [CrossRef]
12. Brook, R.D.; Appel, L.J.; Rubenfire, M.; Ogedegbe, G.; Bisognano, J.D.; Elliott, W.J.; Fuchs, F.D.; Hughes, J.W.; Lackland, D.T.; Staffileno, B.A.; et al. Beyond medications and diet: Alternative approaches to lowering blood pressure: A scientific statement from the american heart association. *Hypertension* **2013**, *61*, 1360–1383. [CrossRef]
13. Stussman, B.J.; Black, L.I.; Barnes, P.M.; Clarke, T.C.; Nahin, R.L. Wellness-related Use of Common Complementary Health Approaches Among Adults: United States, 2012. *Natl. Health Stat. Rep.* **2015**, *85*, 1–12.
14. Rakicevic, M. 27 Meditation Statistics for Your Well-Being in 2023. 2022. Available online: https://disturbmenot.co/meditation-statistics/ (accessed on 29 March 2023).
15. Clarke, T.C.; Barnes, P.M.; Black, L.I.; Stussman, B.J.; Nahin, R.L. *Use of Yoga, Meditation, and Chiropractors Among U.S. Adults Aged 18 and Over*; US Department of Health and Human Services, Centers for Disease Control and Prevention, National Center for Health Statistics: Washington, DC, USA, 2018; pp. 1–8.
16. Zeidan, F.; Johnson, S.K.; Gordon, N.S.; Goolkasian, P. Effects of Brief and Sham Mindfulness Meditation on Mood and Cardiovascular Variables. *J. Altern. Complement. Med.* **2010**, *16*, 867–873. [CrossRef] [PubMed]
17. Hughes, J.W.; Fresco, D.M.; Myerscough, R.; van Dulmen, M.H.M.; Carlson, L.E.; Josephson, R. Randomized controlled trial of mindfulness-based stress reduction for prehypertension. *Psychosom. Med.* **2013**, *75*, 721–728. [CrossRef] [PubMed]
18. Paul-Labrador, M.; Polk, D.; Dwyer, J.H.; Velasquez, I.; Nidich, S.; Rainforth, M.; Schneider, R.; Merz, C.N.B. Effects of a Randomized Controlled Trial of Transcendental Meditation on Components of the Metabolic Syndrome in Subjects With Coronary Heart Disease. *Arch. Intern. Med.* **2006**, *166*, 1218–1224. [CrossRef]
19. McGee, M. Meditation and Psychiatry. *Psychiatry* **2008**, *5*, 28–41.
20. Ray, I.B.; Menezes, A.R.; Malur, P.; E Hiltbold, A.; Reilly, J.P.; Lavie, C.J. Meditation and coronary heart disease: A review of the current clinical evidence. *Ochsner J.* **2014**, *14*, 696–703.
21. Rudlof, M.E.; Šimunić, B.; Steuber, B.; Bartel, T.O.; Neshev, R.; Mächler, P.; Dorr, A.; Picha, R.; Schmid-Zalaudek, K.; Goswami, N. Effects of Meditation on Cardiovascular and Muscular Responses in Patients during Cardiac Rehabilitation: A Randomized Pilot Study. *J. Clin. Med.* **2022**, *11*, 6143. [CrossRef]
22. Chu, P.; A Gotink, R.; Yeh, G.Y.; Goldie, S.J.; Hunink, M.M. The effectiveness of yoga in modifying risk factors for cardiovascular disease and metabolic syndrome: A systematic review and meta-analysis of randomized controlled trials. *Eur. J. Prev. Cardiol.* **2014**, *23*, 291–307. [CrossRef]
23. Cramer, H.; Lauche, R.; Haller, H.; Steckhan, N.; Michalsen, A.; Dobos, G. Effects of yoga on cardiovascular disease risk factors: A systematic review and meta-analysis. *Int. J. Cardiol.* **2014**, *173*, 170–183. [CrossRef]
24. Cooper, M.J.; Aygen, M.M. A Relaxation Technique In the Management of Hypercholesterolemia. *J. Hum. Stress* **1979**, *5*, 24–27. [CrossRef]

25. Anderson, J.W.; Liu, C.; Kryscio, R.J. Blood Pressure Response to Transcendental Meditation: A Meta-analysis. *Am. J. Hypertens.* **2008**, *21*, 310–316. [CrossRef] [PubMed]
26. De, A.; Mondal, S.; Deepeshwar, S. Single Bout of Yoga Practices (Asana) Effect on Low Frequency (LF) of Heart Rate Variability—A Pilot Study. *Int. J. Med. Public Health* **2019**, *9*, 160–163. [CrossRef]
27. Krishna, B.H.; Pal, P.; Pal, G.K.; Balachander, J.; Jayasettiaseelon, E.; Sreekanth, Y.; Gaur, G.S. Effect of Yoga Therapy on Heart Rate, Blood Pressure and Cardiac Autonomic Function in Heart Failure. *J. Clin. Diagn. Res.* **2014**, *8*, 14–16. [CrossRef] [PubMed]
28. Deciuceis, C.; Porteri, E.; Rizzoni, D.; Rizzardi, N.; Paiardi, S.; Boari, G.E.; Miclini, M.; Zani, F.; Muiesan, M.L.; Donato, F.; et al. Structural Alterations of Subcutaneous Small-Resistance Arteries May Predict Major Cardiovascular Events in Patients with Hypertension. *Am. J. Hypertens.* **2007**, *20*, 846–852. [CrossRef]
29. Rizzoni, D.; Porteri, E.; Boari, G.E.; De Ciuceis, C.; Sleiman, I.; Muiesan, M.L.; Castellano, M.; Miclini, M.; Agabiti-Rosei, E. Prognostic Significance of Small-Artery Structure in Hypertension. *Circulation* **2003**, *108*, 2230–2235. [CrossRef]
30. Wong T.Y.; Klein, R.; Sharrett, A.R.; Duncan, B.B.; Couper, D.J.; Klein, B.E.; Hubbard, L.D.; Nieto, F.J.; for the Atherosclerosis Risk in Communities Study. Retinal Arteriolar Diameter and Risk for Hypertension. *Ann. Intern. Med.* **2004**, *140*, 248–255. [CrossRef]
31. Ikram, M.K.; Witteman, J.C.; Vingerling, J.R.; Breteler, M.M.; Hofman, A.; de Jong, P.T. Retinal Vessel Diameters and Risk of Hypertension. *Hypertension* **2006**, *47*, 189–194. [CrossRef]
32. Tanabe, Y.; Kawasaki, R.; Wang, J.J.; Wong, T.Y.; Mitchell, P.; Daimon, M.; Oizumi, T.; Kato, T.; Kawata, S.; Kayama, T.; et al. Retinal Arteriolar Narrowing Predicts 5-Year Risk of Hypertension in Japanese People: The Funagata Study. *Microcirculation* **2010**, *17*, 94–102. [CrossRef]
33. Nguyen, T.T.; Wong, T.Y. Retinal vascular manifestations of metabolic disorders. *Trends Endocrinol. Metab.* **2006**, *17*, 262–268. [CrossRef]
34. Wong, T.Y.; Mitchell, P. Hypertensive Retinopathy. *N. Engl. J. Med.* **2004**, *351*, 2310–2317. [CrossRef]
35. Wong, T.; Mitchell, P. The eye in hypertension. *Lancet* **2007**, *369*, 425–435. [CrossRef] [PubMed]
36. Wang, J.J.; Liew, G.; Klein, R.; Rochtchina, E.; Knudtson, M.D.; Klein, B.E.; Wong, T.Y.; Burlutsky, G.; Mitchell, P. Retinal vessel diameter and cardiovascular mortality: Pooled data analysis from two older populations. *Eur. Hear. J.* **2007**, *28*, 1984–1992. [CrossRef] [PubMed]
37. Wong, T.Y.; Kamineni, A.; Klein, R.; Sharrett, A.R.; Klein, B.E.; Siscovick, D.S.; Cushman, M.; Duncan, B.B. Quantitative Retinal Venular Caliber and Risk of Cardiovascular Disease in Older Persons. *Arch. Intern. Med.* **2006**, *166*, 2388–2394. [CrossRef] [PubMed]
38. Merz, C.N.B.; Dwyer, J.; Nordstrom, C.K.; Walton, K.G.; Salerno, J.W.; Schneider, R.H. Psychosocial Stress and Cardiovascular Disease: Pathophysiological Links. *Behav. Med.* **2002**, *27*, 141–147. [CrossRef]
39. Yusuf, S.; Hawken, S.; Ôunpuu, S.; Dans, T.; Avezum, A.; Lanas, F.; McQueen, M.; Budaj, A.; Pais, P.; Varigos, J.; et al. Effect of potentially modifiable risk factors associated with myocardial infarction in 52 countries (the INTERHEART study): Case-control study. *Lancet* **2004**, *364*, 937–952. [CrossRef]
40. Thabane, L.; Ma, J.; Chu, R.; Cheng, J.; Ismaila, A.; Rios, L.P.; Robson, R.; Thabane, M.; Giangregorio, L.; Goldsmith, C.H. A tutorial on pilot studies: The what, why and how. *BMC Med. Res. Methodol.* **2010**, *10*, 1. [CrossRef]
41. Hopewell, S.; Clarke, M.; Moher, D.; Wager, E.; Middleton, P.; Altman, D.G.; Schulz, K.F.; the CONSORT Group. CONSORT for Reporting Randomized Controlled Trials in Journal and Conference Abstracts: Explanation and Elaboration. *PLoS Med.* **2008**, *5*, e20. [CrossRef]
42. Dinevski, D.; Lučovnik, M.; Žebeljan, I.; Guzelj, D.; Dinevski, I.V.; Saloň, A.; De Boever, P.; Goswami, N. Analysis of Retinal Blood Vessel Diameters in Pregnant Women Practicing Yoga: A Feasibility Study. *Healthcare* **2022**, *10*, 1356. [CrossRef]
43. Everson, F.; De Boever, P.; Nawrot, T.S.; Goswami, N.; Mthethwa, M.; Webster, I.; Martens, D.S.; Mashele, N.; Charania, S.; Kamau, F.; et al. Personal NO_2 and Volatile Organic Compounds Exposure Levels are Associated with Markers of Cardiovascular Risk in Women in the Cape Town Region of South Africa. *Int. J. Environ. Res. Public Health* **2019**, *16*, 2284. [CrossRef]
44. Hosák, L.; Zeman, T.; Studnička, J.; Stepanov, A.; Ustohal, L.; Michalec, M.; Lochman, J.; Jurečka, T.; Sadykov, E.; Goswami, N.; et al. Retinal arteriolar and venular diameters are widened in patients with schizophrenia. *Psychiatry Clin. Neurosci.* **2020**, *74*, 619–621. [CrossRef]
45. Louwies, T.; De Boever, P.; Hasso, R.; Tremblay, M.F.; Xu, D.; Blaber, A.P.; Goswami, N. Retinal blood vessel diameter changes with 60-day head-down bedrest are unaffected by antioxidant nutritional cocktail. *npj Microgravity* **2024**, *10*, 1–7. [CrossRef] [PubMed]
46. Louwies, T.; Panis, L.I.; Alders, T.; Bonné, K.; Goswami, N.; Nawrot, T.S.; Dendale, P.; De Boever, P. Microvascular reactivity in rehabilitating cardiac patients based on measurements of retinal blood vessel diameters. *Microvasc. Res.* **2019**, *124*, 25–29. [CrossRef] [PubMed]
47. Matušková, V.; Zeman, T.; Ewerlingová, L.; Hlinomazová, Z.; Souček, J.; Vlková, E.; Goswami, N.; Balcar, V.J.; Šerý, O. An association of neovascular age-related macular degeneration with polymorphisms of CFH, ARMS2, HTRA1 and C3 genes in Czech population. *Acta Ophthalmol.* **2020**, *98*, e691–e699. [CrossRef] [PubMed]

48. Fabiani, E.; Herc, M.; Simunic, B.; Brix, B.; Loefflers, K.; Weidinger, L.; Zieg, A.; Kastner, P.; Kapel, A.; Goswami, N. Correlation between timed up and go test and skeletal muscle tensiomyography in female nursing home residents. *J. Musculoskelet. Neuronal. Interact.* **2021**, *21*, 247–254.
49. Knudtson, M.D.; Lee, K.E.; Hubbard, L.D.; Wong, T.Y.; Klein, R.; Klein, B.E. Revised formulas for summarizing retinal vessel diameters. *Curr. Eye Res.* **2003**, *27*, 143–149. [CrossRef]
50. Saloň, A.; Çiftci, G.M.; Zubac, D.; Šimunič, B.; Pišot, R.; Narici, M.; Fredriksen, P.M.; Nkeh-Chungag, B.N.; Sourij, H.; Šerý, O.; et al. Retinal venular vessel diameters are smaller during ten days of bed rest. *Sci. Rep.* **2023**, *13*, 19258. [CrossRef]
51. Saloň, A.; Neshev, R.; Teraž, K.; Šimunič, B.; Peskar, M.; Marušič, U.; Pišot, S.; Šlosar, L.; Gasparini, M.; Pišot, R.; et al. A pilot study: Exploring the influence of COVID-19 on cardiovascular physiology and retinal microcirculation. *Microvasc. Res.* **2023**, *150*, 104588. [CrossRef]
52. Saloň, A.; Steuber, B.; Neshev, R.; Schmid-Zalaudek, K.; De Boever, P.; Bergmann, E.; Picha, R.; Fredriksen, P.M.; Nkeh-Chungag, B.N.; Goswami, N. Vascular Responses following Light Therapy: A Pilot Study with Healthy Volunteers. *J. Clin. Med.* **2023**, *12*, 2229. [CrossRef]
53. Saloň, A.; Vladic, N.; Schmid-Zalaudek, K.; Steuber, B.; Hawliczek, A.; Urevc, J.; Bergauer, A.; Pivec, V.; Shankhwar, V.; Goswami, N. Sex Variations in Retinal Microcirculation Response to Lower Body Negative Pressure. *Biology* **2023**, *12*, 1224. [CrossRef]
54. Saloň, A.; De Boever, P.; Goswami, N. Microvascular Changes during Viral Infections: A Systematic Review of Studies Using Retinal Vessel Diameter Assessments. *Biomedicines* **2024**, *12*, 1488. [CrossRef]
55. Saloň, A.; Schmid-Zalaudek, K.; Steuber, B.; Müller, A.; Moser, O.; Alnuaimi, S.; Fredriksen, P.M.; Ngwenchi Nkeh-Chungag, B.; Goswami, N. Acute effects of exercise on macro- and microvasculature in individuals with type 1 diabetes—A secondary outcome analysis. *Front. Endocrinol.* **2024**, *15*, 1406930. [CrossRef] [PubMed]
56. Pinckard, K.; Baskin, K.K.; Stanford, K.I. Effects of Exercise to Improve Cardiovascular Health. *Front. Cardiovasc. Med.* **2019**, *6*, 69. [CrossRef] [PubMed]
57. Fiuza-Luces, C.; Santos-Lozano, A.; Joyner, M.; Carrera-Bastos, P.; Picazo, O.; Zugaza, J.L.; Izquierdo, M.; Ruilope, L.M.; Lucia, A. Exercise benefits in cardiovascular disease: Beyond attenuation of traditional risk factors. *Nat. Rev. Cardiol.* **2018**, *15*, 731–743. [CrossRef] [PubMed]
58. Hambrecht, R.; Wolf, A.; Gielen, S.; Linke, A.; Hofer, J.; Erbs, S.; Schoene, N.; Schuler, G. Effect of Exercise on Coronary Endothelial Function in Patients with Coronary Artery Disease. *N. Engl. J. Med.* **2000**, *342*, 454–460. [CrossRef] [PubMed]
59. Fagard, R.H. Exercise characteristics and the blood pressure response to dynamic physical training. *Med. Sci. Sports Exerc.* **2001**, *33*, S484–S492. [CrossRef]
60. Taylor, R.S.; Brown, A.; Ebrahim, S.; Jolliffe, J.; Noorani, H.; Rees, K.; Skidmore, B.; A Stone, J.; Thompson, D.R.; Oldridge, N. Exercise-based rehabilitation for patients with coronary heart disease: Systematic review and meta-analysis of randomized controlled trials. *Am. J. Med.* **2004**, *116*, 682–692. [CrossRef]
61. Cornelissen, V.A.; Fagard, R.H. Effects of Endurance Training on Blood Pressure, Blood Pressure–Regulating Mechanisms, and Cardiovascular Risk Factors. *Hypertension* **2005**, *46*, 667–675. [CrossRef]
62. Murugesan, R.; Govindarajulu, N.; Bera, T.K. Effect of selected yogic practices on the management of hypertension. *Indian J. Physiol. Pharmacol.* **2000**, *44*, 207–210.
63. Pal, A.; Srivastava, N.; Tiwari, S.; Verma, N.; Narain, V.; Agrawal, G.; Natu, S.; Kumar, K. Effect of yogic practices on lipid profile and body fat composition in patients of coronary artery disease. *Complement. Ther. Med.* **2011**, *19*, 122–127. [CrossRef]
64. Bharshankar, J.R.; Bharshankar, R.N.; Deshpande, V.N.; Kaore, S.B.; Gosavi, G.B. Effect of yoga on cardiovascular system in subjects above 40 years. *Indian J. Physiol. Pharmacol.* **2003**, *47*, 202–206.
65. Meles, E.; Giannattasio, C.; Failla, M.; Gentile, G.; Capra, A.; Mancia, G. Nonpharmacologic treatment of hypertension by respiratory exercise in the home setting. *Am. J. Hypertens.* **2004**, *17*, 370–374. [CrossRef] [PubMed]
66. Dillbeck, M.C.; Orme-Johnson, D.W. Physiological differences between transcendental meditation and rest. *Am. Psychol.* **1987**, *42*, 879–881. [CrossRef]
67. Schneider, R.H.; Staggers, F.; Alexander, C.N.; Sheppard, W.; Rainforth, M.; Kondwani, K.; Smith, S.; King, C.G. A Randomized Controlled Trial of Stress Reduction for Hypertension in Older African Americans. *Hypertension* **1995**, *26*, 820–827. [CrossRef] [PubMed]
68. Rainforth, M.V.; Schneider, R.H.; Nidich, S.I.; Gaylord-King, C.; Salerno, J.W.; Anderson, J.W. Stress reduction programs in patients with elevated blood pressure: A systematic review and meta-analysis. *Curr. Hypertens. Rep.* **2007**, *9*, 520–528. [CrossRef]

Journal of
Clinical Medicine

MDPI

Review

Mitochondrial Bioenergetics and Cardiac Rehabilitation: Bridging Basic Science and Clinical Practice

Angela Dziedzic [1], Klaudia Marek [2], Piotr Niebrzydowski [3], Dominika Szalewska [3,4,*], Patrycja Nowak [1] and Elżbieta Miller [2,*]

[1] Department of General Biochemistry, Faculty of Biology and Environmental Protection, University of Lodz, Pomorska 141/143, 90-236 Lodz, Poland; angela.dziedzic@biol.uni.lodz.pl (A.D.); patrycja.nowak5@edu.uni.lodz.pl (P.N.)
[2] Department of Neurological Rehabilitation, Medical University of Lodz, Milionowa 14, 93-113 Lodz, Poland; klaudia.marek@umed.lodz.pl
[3] Clinic of Rehabilitation, University Clinical Center in Gdansk, al. Zwycięstwa 30, 80-219 Gdansk, Poland; pniebrzydowski@uck.gda.pl
[4] Division of Rehabilitation Medicine, Faculty of Health Sciences, Medical University of Gdansk, al. Zwycięstwa 30, 80-219 Gdansk, Poland
* Correspondence: dominika.szalewska@gumed.edu.pl (D.S.); elzbieta.dorota.miller@umed.lodz.pl (E.M.)

Abstract: Cardiovascular diseases (CVDs) are the leading cause of global morbidity and mortality, underscoring the necessity of long-term secondary prevention strategies such as comprehensive cardiac rehabilitation (CR). CR is a clinically validated, cost-effective intervention that mitigates cardiovascular risk, improves functional capacity, and enhances patient prognosis. Emerging evidence emphasizes the pivotal role of mitochondrial bioenergetics in mediating the systemic benefits of exercise-based CR, particularly through mechanisms involving mitochondrial biogenesis, dynamics, and mitophagy. This review synthesizes molecular insights with clinical guidelines by evaluating four national CR guidelines—from Poland, France, the United States, and Portugal—alongside a comprehensive recommendation issued by the European Society of Cardiology (ESC). The analysis focused on key components of CR, including exercise modalities (aerobic, resistance, and high-intensity interval training) and prescription parameters such as frequency, intensity, and duration. Only guidelines fulfilling predefined inclusion criteria with complete and detailed data were included; documents lacking essential information were excluded from the final synthesis.

Keywords: cardiac rehabilitation; exercise; cardiovascular disease; mitochondrial bioenergetics

1. Introduction

Cardiovascular diseases (CVDs) persist as the predominant cause of morbidity and mortality globally, despite notable advancements in acute medical and interventional therapies. Consequently, long-term management strategies, particularly those aimed at lifestyle modification and functional recovery, have become integral to secondary prevention efforts. Among these strategies, comprehensive cardiac rehabilitation (CR) has emerged as a critical intervention, demonstrating significant efficacy in reducing the incidence of recurrent cardiovascular events, enhancing quality of life, and improving overall prognosis in patients with CVDs [1]. As articulated by Jegier et al. (2021), CR should not be considered a mere adjunctive therapy; rather, it is a clinically validated, cost-effective, and multidimensional intervention that significantly contributes to cardiovascular risk mitigation and long-term patient outcomes [2]. Despite the robust clinical evidence supporting the efficacy of CR, the underlying physiological mechanisms—particularly at the cellular and molecular levels—warrant further elucidation [3]. Recent research increasingly emphasizes the role of mitochondrial function and bioenergetics in mediating the cardiovascular and systemic benefits associated with exercise-based rehabilitation. Mitochondria, often referred to as the bioenergetic powerhouses of the cell, are pivotal regulators of energy metabolism, redox signaling, and cellular adaptation to oxidative stress. Their dynamic responses to physical exercise not only affect skeletal muscle function but also play a critical role in cardiac metabolism, vascular health, and the regulation of systemic inflammatory processes, all of which are essential to the rehabilitative approach [4,5]. This review aims to synthesize insights from basic mitochondrial biology with clinical rehabilitation medicine and cardiology by investigating how exercise-induced mitochondrial adaptations enhance the efficacy of CR. It explores evidence-based recommendations and guidelines pertaining to CR in different countries and current understanding of mitochondrial biogenesis, dynamics, and mitophagy in exercise physiology and its protective role in mitigating pathophysiological conditions in cardiological patients. By combining molecular and physiological research with clinical results, we aim to create a framework that explains the underlying mechanisms of CR and informs future therapeutic strategies.

2. Materials and Methods

Databases and publishers were used to search for CR recommendations and guidelines. The electronic databases PubMed, Medline, and ScienceDirect were searched extensively. A systematic review was conducted manually. The following keyword search was used: CR recommendations. The following information was expected: (1) main recommendations and details of the CR program (e.g., risk factor prevention, patient education, physical activity suggested, safety, health monitoring); (2) types of exercise used in the CR program (resistance, aerobic, HIIT); and (3) frequency, intensity, duration, and details of specific forms of training.

In the absence of relevant information (no list of types of training, no main recommendations), the study was excluded due to insufficient data. Five published recommendations and advice on CR were qualified. Four were country-specific: Poland, France, the US, and Portugal. One article was about European recommendations. Four recommendations were published in the English language. One article from Poland was published in Polish. Organizations that provided recommendations and advice were the following: (1) Poland—Section of Cardiac Rehabilitation and Exercise Physiology of the Polish Cardiac Society; (2) France—French Society of Cardiology, Groupe Exercise Rehabilitation Sports—Prevention (GERS-P); (3) the US—American Heart Association (AHA), American Association of Cardiovascular and Pulmonary Rehabilitation (AACVPR); (4) Portugal—Portuguese Society of Cardiology (PSC); and (5) Europe—European Society of Cardiology (ESC). Articles with incomplete data and recommendations were excluded and not considered in the review. Therefore, only five studies that met all requirements were accepted and included in our quality synthesis (Figure 1).

This review considers published recommendations from the past nine years. This systematic review aims to answer the following questions: What are the latest recommendations for CR in different countries?

This review considers published recommendations from the past nine years. This systematic review aims to answer the following questions: What are the latest recommendations for cardiac rehabilitation in different countries?

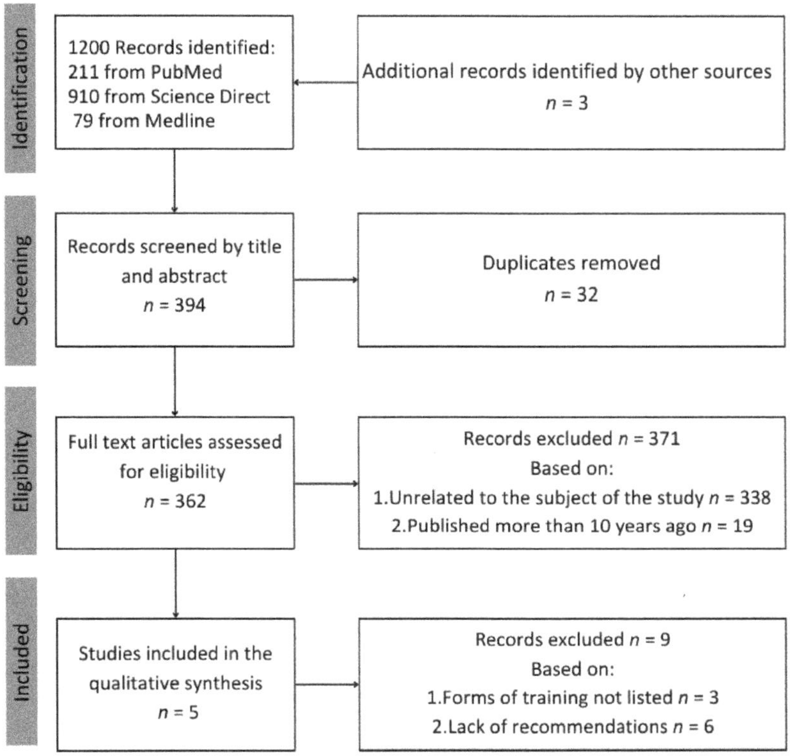

Figure 1. Flowchart of study selection.

3. Results

CR is a complex process offered to patients who have been diagnosed with heart disease. The intervention includes, but is not limited to, elements of health education, advice on cardiovascular risk factors, dietary advice, physical activity, and stress management [6–8]. Evidence from a number of published systematic reviews and meta-analyses suggests that CR reduces mortality, recurrent cardiac events, and hospitalization, and improves exercise capacity, quality of life, and mental health. Recommendations for the use of CR are increasing and it is now recommended in international guidelines [6,9].

Specific guidelines for CR were collected and compared, distinguishing the following aspects (Table 1):

1. Breakdown of rehabilitation into stages/phases
2. Psychological support
3. Training plan
4. Multidisciplinary team
5. Patient education
6. Health monitoring
7. Sexual activity
8. Pharmacotherapy
9. Nutritional counselling
10. Daily living and return to work

Table 1. Comparing key factors in CR programs around the world.

Factor/Organization	Cardiac Rehabilitation and Exercise Physiology Section of the Polish Cardiac Society 2021, Poland [2].	French Society of Cardiology, Groupe Exercise Rehabilitation Sports—Prevention, 2023, France [10].	American College of Cardiology, American Heart Association, JACC Expert Panel, 2024, US [11].	Portuguese Society of Cardiology, 2018, Portugal [12].	European Association for Cardiovascular Prevention and Rehabilitation, 2016, Europe [13].
Breakdown of rehabilitation into stages/phases	**Stage I—Early (in-hospital) rehabilitation:** Begins during hospitalization after a cardiovascular event and continues until the patient is discharged from the hospital. Carried out in the intensive care unit, post-operative care unit, cardiology, internal medicine, or CR. **Stage II—Early rehabilitation (outpatient/inpatient):** Can be performed entirely in the inpatient setting, in a center/day unit (outpatient), or as a hybrid cardiac telerehabilitation (HCTR). Inpatient form for patients at high cardiovascular risk, with complications after treatment of acute coronary syndromes (ACSs), cardiac surgery, or percutaneous coronary intervention (PCI), with stable, advanced heart failure (HF) in NYHA class III–IV, immediately after heart transplantation (HT), or for those who, for logistical reasons, cannot participate in rehabilitation programs. **Stage III—Late (outpatient) rehabilitation:** Implemented in a day/outpatient setting Includes health education program for patient and family. Continuous monitoring based on individual needs and cardiac risk profile. Stage III continues for the rest of the patient's life	No specific breakdown	No specific breakdown	**Hospital Phase I:** begins 24–48 h after a patient is stabilized following an acute event. Includes early mobilization, low-intensity exercise and education. **Early Post-Discharge Phase II:** begins within two weeks of hospital discharge or after diagnosis. It can be conducted in the hospital, a specialized CR center, or in the patient's home. Includes individualized exercise, education, and lifestyle modification. **Long-term Phase III:** begins after Phase II and continues for the rest of the patient's life. Aims at long-term maintenance of rehabilitation effects, control of risk factors, and monitoring of health status.	No specific breakdown

Table 1. *Cont.*

Factor/Organization	Cardiac Rehabilitation and Exercise Physiology Section of the Polish Cardiac Society 2021, Poland [2].	French Society of Cardiology, Groupe Exercise Rehabilitation Sports—Prevention, 2023, France [10].	American College of Cardiology, American Heart Association, JACC Expert Panel, 2024, US [11].	Portuguese Society of Cardiology, 2018, Portugal [12].	European Association for Cardiovascular Prevention and Rehabilitation, 2016, Europe [13].
Psychological suport	Assessment of mental status and development of an individual psychological care plan. Psychological assistance, especially for sleep disorders, anxiety, depression, mental health deterioration, and reduced quality of life.	Psychosocial assessment at the beginning of the rehabilitation process. Access to psychologist during rehabilitation. Mental status monitoring.	Detailed psychological assessment, including depression, perceived stress, anxiety, sexual dysfunction, anger, loneliness, social isolation, and problematic substance abuse. Psychological interventions and patient education.	Assessment and psychological interventions to reduce stress, anxiety, and depression.	Assessment of psychosocial factors. Specialized psychological interventions.
Training plan	Individualized exercise program for each patient. The patient must be in a stable clinical condition to begin training. Aerobic endurance training involving large muscle groups—3 days per week/day. Resistance training—2 times a week on non-consecutive days of the week Duration of exercise: 20–30 min minimum (45–60 min preferred) per session. Training intensity should be based on individual exercise tolerance and cardiovascular risk. Train according to the FITT rule (frequency, intensity, time-duration, type of exercise). Energy expenditure during exercise of 1000–2000 kcal/week.	Individual exercise program for each patient Frequency: 3–6 times a week Duration: Warm-up: 5–10 min Exercise proper: 20–45 min —Cooling down: at least 5 min. Type: Aerobic Continuous at moderate intensity Interval Resistance. Respiratory: The program should last at least 12 weeks.	Individualized plan, updated every 30 days with health assessment Aerobic training—3–5 days a week, Moderate intensity (40–59%) and high intensity (60–89%) with effort assessment, 20–60 min. Resistance training—2–3 days a week, on non-consecutive days, 10–15 repetitions with 40–60% 1-RM load (maximum load that can be lifted once) with effort assessment.	**Early Phase I**—Early mobilization and low-intensity exercises. Intensity: Determined by the subjective feeling of exertion as assessed by the Borg scale, without exceeding the resting heart rate by 20–30 beats per minute, depending on the patient's clinical condition. **Phase II** early after hospital discharge. Individualized training program including aerobic and resistance exercises Duration: 8–12 weeks.	Regular physical activity is recommended as a lifelong lifestyle for all men and women, including ≥150 min/week of moderate-intensity activity or ≥75 min/week of vigorous-intensity activity. Aerobic exercise. Resistance training—2–3 sets of 8–12 repetitions at an intensity of 60–80% of 1 repetition performed at a person's 1-ROM, with a frequency of ≥2 days per week. Neuromotor training.

Table 1. *Cont.*

Factor/Organization	Cardiac Rehabilitation and Exercise Physiology Section of the Polish Cardiac Society 2021, Poland [2].	French Society of Cardiology, Groupe Exercise Rehabilitation Sports—Prevention, 2023, France [10].	American College of Cardiology, American Heart Association, JACC Expert Panel, 2024, US [11].	Portuguese Society of Cardiology, 2018, Portugal [12].	European Association for Cardiovascular Prevention and Rehabilitation, 2016, Europe [13].
Multidisciplinary team	Physician, physiotherapist, nurse, radiology technician, psychologist, nutritionist, rehabilitation management specialist.	Physician, nurse, physiotherapist, social worker, nutritionist, psychologist, physical activity trainer.	Physician, nurse, physiotherapist, nutritionist, respiratory therapist, behavioral health expert.	Cardiologist, physiotherapist, rehabilitation nurse, nutritionist, psychologist, psychiatrist, and other specialists as needed by the patient.	Physician, physiotherapist, nurse, nutritionist, pharmacist, sports medicine expert.
Patient education	Risk factor modification: dyslipidemia, hypertension, diabetes, obesity, smoking, and physical inactivity. Healthy lifestyle and physical activity, pharmacotherapy, symptom self-management, and stress management.	Modification of cardiovascular risk factors. Nutrition education. Physical activity education.	Modification of risk factors: physical activity, diet, mental health, sleep, avoidance of unhealthy behaviors (smoking, alcohol, drug abuse).	Counseling on healthy lifestyle, diet, exercise, returning to work, and managing stress and anxiety. Maintaining long-term control of cardiovascular risk factors and adherence to medications and healthy lifestyles.	Disease knowledge. Modification of risk factors—smoking, unhealthy diet, physical inactivity, hypertension, hyperlipidemia, and diabetes. Stress management education.
Health monitoring	Observation of the patient. Assessment of clinical condition before each training—measurement of blood pressure and heart rate. Performing tests: ECG, exercise test, Cardiopulmonary Exercise Test (CPET), 6-min walk test (6-MWT), laboratory tests, transthoracic echocardiography (TTE).	Regular review of risk factors. Monitoring: heart rate and oxygen saturation during exercise. Physical fitness assessment: 6-min walk test, Cardiopulmonary Exercise Test (CPET), ankle–arm index measurement, arterial echo-doppler, Holter-EKG, ambulatory blood pressure monitoring, overnight polygraphy, pulmonary function testing.	Monitor blood pressure and ECG during exercise, especially in high-risk patients. Evaluate progress and adjust exercise plan based on patient response and results achieved.	Risk factor control: Interventions to control hypertension, diabetes, hyperlipidemia, obesity, and smoking. Medical evaluation: Assessment of medical history, risk factors, functional status, and test results (ECG, blood tests, echocardiography).	Monitoring of risk factors: BMI, cholesterol, blood pressure, smoking. Monitoring treatment.

Table 1. *Cont.*

Factor/Organization	Cardiac Rehabilitation and Exercise Physiology Section of the Polish Cardiac Society 2021, Poland [2].	French Society of Cardiology, Groupe Exercise Rehabilitation Sports—Prevention, 2023, France [10].	American College of Cardiology, American Heart Association, JACC Expert Panel, 2024, US [11].	Portuguese Society of Cardiology, 2018, Portugal [12].	European Association for Cardiovascular Prevention and Rehabilitation, 2016, Europe [13].
Sexual activity	Information on how to implement physical activity and return to sexual activity is included in patient education.	Therapy related to sexual activity must be offered to both men and women, taking into account the psychological dimension and individual wishes of the patients. Determine the cause of the difficulty: may be due to the disease itself, comorbidities, and medications used (beta-blockers, diuretics, antihypertensives). Possible use of phosphodiesterase inhibitors. Patients with unstable cardiovascular disease or symptoms should not engage in sexual activity until their condition has stabilized.	Psychosocial assessment, including sexual dysfunction. Psychosocial interventions—sex and intimacy education and counseling.	Patient education includes counseling on returning to sexual activity	Possible occurrence of erectile dysfunction due to a cardiovascular event in the future. Modification of risk factors: hypercholesterolemia, hypertension, insulin resistance and diabetes, smoking, obesity, metabolic syndrome, sedentary lifestyle, and depression. Recommend pharmacotherapy.
Pharmacotherapy	Analysis of existing pharmacotherapy with the possibility of its modification depending on clinical condition and in accordance with general recommendations. Pharmacotherapy education.	Monitor drug therapy: Optimize drug therapy, including anticoagulant therapy, and monitor potassium levels and kidney function after each change in therapy.	Evaluate current treatment and modify if necessary. Patient education—importance of adherence to medication recommendations.	Optimization of pharmacotherapy (phase II). Pharmacologic compliance education.	Optimization of pharmacotherapy. Adherence to recommendations. A multicomponent pill (polypill) may be considered to improve adherence to prescribed pharmacotherapy.

Table 1. *Cont.*

Factor/Organization	Cardiac Rehabilitation and Exercise Physiology Section of the Polish Cardiac Society 2021, Poland [2].	French Society of Cardiology, Groupe Exercise Rehabilitation Sports—Prevention, 2023, France [10].	American College of Cardiology, American Heart Association, JACC Expert Panel, 2024, US [11].	Portuguese Society of Cardiology, 2018, Portugal [12].	European Association for Cardiovascular Prevention and Rehabilitation, 2016, Europe [13].
Nutritional counselling	Recognize and counteract the effects of malnutrition. Education about healthy nutrition by a nutritionist.	Mediterranean diet. Eating at least 5 servings of fruits and vegetables per day. Limiting the intake of salt and products containing simple sugars. Avoiding processed foods. Nutrition education.	Diet evaluation. Discussion of eating habits. Nutrition education. Individualized nutrition plan.	Dietary counseling, including assessment and advice from dietitians.	Individual dietary recommendations. Avoiding overeating. When following a healthy diet, supplements are not recommended. Limit salt intake. Mediterranean diet. Nutrition education.

Abbreviations: HCTR—Hybrid comprehensive telerehabilitation, ACS—Acute coronary syndrome, HF—Heart failure, HT—Heart transplantation, PCI—Percutaneous coronary intervention, FITT—frequency, intensity, time-duration, type of exercise, CPET—Cardiopulmonary Exercise Test.

According to recommendations from Poland and Portugal, CR is divided into three phases. The first phase is early inpatient rehabilitation, the second phase is outpatient rehabilitation once the patient's condition has stabilized, and the third phase is late outpatient rehabilitation, which lasts for the rest of the patient's life. Psychological support for the patient is an important part of the rehabilitation process, especially for patients with adjustment disorders, depression, or anxiety. Psychological support is recommended by all the organizations involved in the review. The detailed presentation of a plan for resistance training, aerobic training, and HIIT is recommended by all countries. The Portuguese Society of Cardiology identified and recommended the above forms of physical activity, but did not elaborate on the intensity, frequency, type, and monitoring of the patient's health and safety during training.

The need for a multidisciplinary team in the program was raised by all the organizations making recommendations. The team should consist of physicians specialized in physical and rehabilitation medicine (PRM), cardiologists, physiotherapists, nurses, dieticians, psychologists, psychiatrists, radiographers, a pharmacist, and other specialists as required by the patient's needs. Patient education focuses on elements of risk factor modification, stress management situations, healthy eating, pharmacotherapy, and physical activity. Health monitoring and functional assessment form the basis of a proper CR process. Tests that should be monitored include ECG, blood pressure, echo, stress test, blood tests, and exercise tests. All organizations address the issue of sexual activity after a cardiovascular event. Therapy related to sexual activity must be offered to both men and women, taking into account the psychological dimension and the individual wishes of the patients. The cause of the disorder affecting the patient's sexual life must be identified. Patients with known unstable cardiovascular disease or symptoms should not engage in sexual activity until their condition has stabilized. If the effects of therapy are not successful, pharmacotherapies should be considered after consultation with a doctor.

All recommendations emphasize evaluation of current treatment and modification with the aim of optimization. Patients should be counseled about medication use and adherence. The European recommendations suggest that a polypill should be considered to improve adherence to prescribed medication in patients with difficulties. Recommendations on dietary advice include an individualized dietary plan for patients, which should be based on the Mediterranean diet. Salt, processed foods, and sweets should be limited and overeating should be avoided [14]. In the US recommendations, there was an emphasis on methods to protect against extreme heat. Extreme heat exposure can be particularly hazardous for cardiac patients. Aerobic endurance exercise is an essential part of a cardiac patient's training plan [1]. Until recently, resistance exercise was considered unsafe due to the sudden increase in blood pressure and heart rate [15]. Evidence suggests that resistance exercise can be performed safely in cardiac patients up to 90% of 1 repetition maximum (1RM) [16]. The combination of aerobic and resistance exercise has a positive effect on muscular performance and strength [17]. High-intensity interval training, which combines repetitive high-intensity activity with periods of rest or active recovery at lower intensity, is becoming increasingly common in CR recommendations. The increased interest in this type of training is due to positive results in patients with chronic heart disease. In addition, studies have shown improvements in cardiovascular and metabolic function [18]. CR programs in Europe are characterized by low dropout rates among patients and short average wait times for rehabilitation after a myocardial infarction. The state ensures the smooth running of the program through public funding [19]. The approach and recommendations for specific recommended forms of exercise, such as resistance training, aerobic exercise, and high-intensity interval training, were compared [Table 2].

Table 2. Recommendations for resistance, aerobic, and high-intensity interval training in cardiac patients.

Author, Year, Country	Resistance Training	Aerobic Training	High-Intensity Interval Training
Jegier, 2021, Poland [2].	• From stage II of rehabilitation, after at least one week of well-tolerated and supervised endurance exercise. • Frequency of exercise: 2 times per week on non-consecutive days of the week. • Exercise intensity: 30–70% 1 repetition maximum (1RM)—the load at which a maximum of 1 full repetition can be performed for the upper extremities and 40–80% 1RM for the lower extremities, with 12–15 repetitions in each set. • Type of exercises: Muscle strength training—resistance exercises and general development exercises, including those to improve flexibility, balance, and inspiratory muscle training. • Training planning in patients with heart failure (HF): Initially, training intensity should be no more than 30% 1-RM, 5–10 repetitions, 2–3 sessions per week, 1–3 cycles per session. • Then gradually increase to 30–40% 1RM, 12–25 repetitions, 2–3 sessions per week, 1 cycle per session. • If tolerance is good, loads of 40–60% 1RM, 8–15 repetitions, 2–3 sessions per week with 1 cycle per session can be used. • Determine the time relationship between muscle contraction (1–3 s) and muscle rest (e.g., 1:2 ratio).	• Physical training should be prepared according to the FITT rule. • Physical training in CR should provide exercise energy consumption of 1000–2000 kcal/week. • Frequency of training: at least 3 days a week, preferably daily. • Moderate intensity: 45–59% of peak oxygen uptake (VO_2 peak), 50–70% of peak load expressed in watt units [W] above first ventilatory threshold (Wpeak), 55–69% of peak HR (HRpeak), 40–59% of heart rate reserve (HR reserve), 4–6 METs (metabolic equivalent of task) or 12–14 points on Borg's 6–20-point interval-form exercise severity perception scale. • Duration of training session: At least 20–30 min, 45–60 min preferred per session. • Type of training, type of physical exercise: Aerobic efforts (marching, trotting, cycling, swimming, rowing, dancing), muscle strength training—resistance exercises—and general development exercises, including those that improve flexibility, balance, and exercise the inspiratory muscles. • Form of training: Training can be done in interval or continuous form.	• Acceptable • For patients with heart failure (HF), interval endurance exercise involves periods (10 s to 4 min) of moderate- to high-intensity exercise (50–100% of maximal exercise capacity) interspersed with periods (1–3 min) of very low-intensity exercise or rest. • Heart transplant (HT) patients: For heart transplant patients, exercise intensity during aerobic training should be low initially (<50% VO_2 peak, 10% below anaerobic threshold or <50% peak workload) and gradually increased. • The decision to incorporate HIIT should always be made on an individual basis, taking into account the patient's clinical condition, exercise tolerance, and cardiovascular risk. Medical evaluation and appropriate monitoring are required prior to initiating such training.

Table 2. *Cont.*

Author, Year, Country	Resistance Training	Aerobic Training	High-Intensity Interval Training
	• Patients after cardiac surgery: Exercise that may interfere with sternal fusion should be avoided. Upper body stretching exercises can be introduced 6 weeks after surgery. • Patients with left ventricular assist devices (VADs): Resistance training, especially of the lower extremity muscles, is indicated. Exercises that are not recommended include running, rowing, crossfit, abdominal exercises, exercises performed with both arms above the head such as weight-lifting, swimming. • Heart transplant patients: to increase muscle mass, bone density, and counteract the adverse effects of immunotherapy.	• Exercise models: Different models (A, B, C, or D) of physical exercise can be implemented in each stage of CR, depending on exercise tolerance and risk of cardiovascular events. • Continuous endurance exercise (for patients with HF). Patients with severely impaired exercise capacity should start with short, low-intensity bouts of 5–10 min and gradually increase to 30–45–60 min, 3–5 times per week, increasing the intensity over time. • Interval endurance exercise (for patients with HF). Periods (10 s to 4 min) of moderate or high intensity exercise (50–100% of peak exercise capacity) are interspersed with periods (1–3 min) of very low intensity exercise or rest. Typically, an exercise session consists of the four phases described above, preceded by 5–10 min of warm-up and followed by 5–10 min of recovery. • Heart transplant patients: exercise intensity during aerobic training should be low at first (<50% VO_2 peak, 10% below anaerobic threshold or <50% of peak workload) and gradually increased.	

Table 2. *Cont.*

Author, Year, Country	Resistance Training	Aerobic Training	High-Intensity Interval Training
Bigot, 2024, France [10].	• Frequency: resistance training should be performed 2–3 times per week. • The maximum load per repetition (1RM) should be assessed. Assessing the strength of large muscle groups is recommended to guide resistance training. • Intensity: Resistance training should be performed at an intensity of 30–70% 1RM for the upper body and 40–80% 1RM for the lower body. • Initially, 10–15 repetitions per set are recommended, with the possibility of increasing the load as the rehabilitation program progresses. • Recent studies suggest that higher intensities (70% 1-RM, 3–10 repetitions) are preferred over more repetitions. • Session duration: Training sessions should last at least 20–30 min (preferably 45–60 min). • Progression: Progress in resistance training should be monitored using the OMNI-RES scale, on which patients rate perceived load from 0 (very easy) to 10 (very hard).	• The training protocol uses continuous and/or interval intensity exercises. Interval training is particularly useful for patients with the lowest fitness levels. • Frequency: Should take place at a frequency of 3–6 times per week. Session structure: Each session should include: • A warm-up lasting 5–10 min. • Main part (exercise period) lasting 20–45 min. • Calming (rest period) lasting a minimum of 5 min. • Intensity is best determined by load and heart rate at the VT1 ventilation threshold. • If VT1 data is not available, intensity should be set at 40–59% of peak VO_2. • You can also use Karvonen's formula to calculate target heart rate: exercise heart rate = resting heart rate + (heart rate reserve × K). • K = 0.6 for patients without chronotropic-negative drugs (beta-blockers). • K = 0.8 for patients taking chronotropic-negative drugs. • Interval training: combines low-impact aerobics phases with more intense phases that result in lactate production. • Intensity should take into account ventilatory thresholds (VT1 and VT2).	• Intensive phases should take place at 70–80% of peak VO_2, 75–90% of maximum heart rate, or a Borg score of 14–16. • HIIT may be particularly useful for patients with the lowest fitness levels. • During HIIT, intensity should take into account ventilation thresholds (VT1 and VT2). • The intensity can be modified during the program, depending on cardiovascular and muscular tolerance, as well as the patient's psychological progress, guided by the Borg scale. • Safe for patients following myocardial infarction. • Use caution and monitor patients for symptoms. • In patients with heart failure (HF), HIIT training has benefits in terms of quality of life (QoL), recovery of autonomy, and reduction in rehospitalizations, with improvements in exercise capacity similar to those seen in patients with reduced ejection fraction. • HIIT is effective and safe if the exercises are properly adjusted, the intensity is gradually increased, and the patient is regularly monitored for signs of decompensation.

Table 2. *Cont.*

Author, Year, Country	Resistance Training	Aerobic Training	High-Intensity Interval Training
		• Intense phases should occur at 70–80% of peak VO_2, 75–90% of maximum heart rate or a Borg score of 14–16. • Session duration: Sessions should last a minimum of 20–30 min and preferably 45–60 min. • Progression: Intensity may be modified throughout the program depending on cardiovascular and muscular tolerance, as well as the patient's psychological progress, guided by the Borg scale.	
Brown, US, 2024 [11].	• Frequency: 2–3 days a week, on non-consecutive days. • Intensity: 10–15 repetitions, 40–60% of maximum load per repetition (1RM). • Rating of perceived exertion 11–13 on the Borg scale (6–20) • 10–15 repetitions with a load that is 40–60% of your maximum one-repetition effort (1RM), or 11–13 reps on the Borg Scale (6–20). • Time: 1–3 sets, 8–10 different exercises targeting major muscle groups. • Use equipment that is safe and comfortable for the person (bands, machines). • You can use weight machines, free weights, elastic bands or your own body weight.	• Frequency: 3–5 days per week. Stable and able-bodied individuals should be encouraged to do additional exercise at home on days they do not attend CR, aiming to exercise $\geq$ 5 days per week to meet federal physical activity guidelines. Intensity: • Moderate: 40–59% of heart rate reserve. This corresponds to 12 or 13 on the Borg scale (6–20). • High: 60–89% of heart rate reserve. This corresponds to 14–17 on the Borg scale (6–20). • Exercise intensity should be less than 10 beats/min from the heart rate at which symptoms such as angina, drop or plateau in SBP, SBP > 240 mm Hg, DBP > 110 mm Hg, ECG changes, signs of myocardial ischemia, or other symptoms of exercise intolerance occur.	• Safe to use. • Extreme high frequency exercise is not recommended for heart patients. Exercise intensity should be carefully and gradually increased, taking into account the patient's individual abilities and health status. • Intensity: short periods of high-intensity exercise and with periods of rest or low-intensity exercise. • Perform a graded exercise test to objectively determine peak oxygen uptake and target heart rate ranges and to consider ischemic thresholds, intensities associated with abnormal blood pressure response, deviations, symptoms, or arrhythmias.

Table 2. *Cont.*

Author, Year, Country	Resistance Training	Aerobic Training	High-Intensity Interval Training
	• Progression: when the upper limit of repetitions is comfortably reached, increase the load by about 5% or use a resistance band with more tension. • During remote training sessions, it is important that the patient masters proper exercise and breathing technique (exhaling during muscle contraction and inhaling during relaxation) to maintain safety. • With time constraints at rehabilitation centers, focus on multi-joint exercises (e.g., rowing, chest presses).	• Borg scale: You can use the Borg perceived exertion scale (scale 6–20: moderate 12–13 and vigorous 14–16; scale 0–10: moderate 3–4 and vigorous 5–7) to interpret a patient's exertion. • Duration: 20–60 min, including warm-up and cool-down. Length can be increased by 1–5 min per session until target length is reached. • Type: Treadmill, cycling, orbiter, rowing, stair climbing, arm/leg ergometry, stepper and others. It is important to include walking, as it is the main form of physical activity performed throughout the day. Other modalities should also be encouraged, especially those that include upper body exercises, if tolerated. • Volume: The volume (frequency × intensity × time) completed per session and each week should be assessed. This can be expressed in calories or MET × min of activity. • Progression: increase one element (frequency, intensity, duration, type) at a time. • Increase duration by 1–5 min per session until the target duration is reached. • Increase intensity after reaching the target duration. • Increases in intensity of 5–10% are usually well tolerated.	

Table 2. *Cont.*

Author, Year, Country	Resistance Training	Aerobic Training	High-Intensity Interval Training
Abreu, 2018, Portugal [12].	• Strength training is recommended in phases II and III of CR. • Before beginning strength training, the patient should undergo a medical evaluation and fitness assessment to identify potential risks and determine the appropriate level of intensity.	• In phase II, aerobic training of 20–45 min or 30–60 min (Phase III) is recommended at a frequency of 3–5 times per week (Phase II) or 2–5 times per week (Phase III). • Individual training program. • Physical fitness assessment, including exercise testing, is mandatory in phases II and III, unless the patient is unable to perform such testing. • Contraindications to aerobic exercise, such as unstable coronary artery disease, acute heart failure, severe arrhythmias, and other serious clinical conditions, should be considered.	• No specific breakdown.
Piepoli, 2016, Europe [13].	• Training should target major muscle groups and include movements involving multiple joints or complex movements. • Frequency: Training should occur at a frequency of $\geq$ 2 days per week. • Series and repetitions: For each training session, 2–3 series of 8–12 repetitions are suggested. • Intensity: should be 60–80% of the value of 1 repetition performed with the maximum load for a person (1RM; the maximum load that can be taken only once). • Elderly and untrained: In elderly and very untrained people, it is suggested to start with 1 series of 10–15 repetitions with an intensity level of 60–70% of 1RM	• Frequency: physical activity should be used at a frequency of $\geq$ 3–5 sessions per week, and preferably daily. • Duration: We recommend $\geq$30 min per day for 5 days per week of moderate-intensity PA (i.e., 150 min per week) or 15 min per day for 5 days per week of intense PA (75 min per week), or a combination of both in sessions of $\geq$10 min each. Shorter exercise sessions (i.e., <10 min) may be appropriate, especially in very untrained individuals. Longer duration exercise, 40 and 60–90 min per day, respectively, has been suggested for lipid control or weight maintenance. • Intensity: moderate to high intensity aerobic exercise should be recommended.	• In selected stable patients, high-intensity interval training may produce even greater improvements in peak VO_2. • Need to assess clinical status: Prior to initiating any exercise training program, including HIIT, it is necessary to assess clinical and functional status. A comprehensive action sequence diagram has been proposed.

Table 2. *Cont.*

Author, Year, Country	Resistance Training	Aerobic Training	High-Intensity Interval Training
	• Graduation of intensity: For the elderly and very untrained, it is suggested to start with 1 series of 10–15 repetitions at an intensity level of 60–70% of 1RM1. Gradually increasing the load is key to avoiding injury and overtraining. • Warming up before exercise and cooling down after exercise can prevent the occurrence of injuries and adverse cardiac events.	• Examples of aerobic activity: cycling or walking, household chores, gardening, work activities, Nordic walking, hiking, jogging, running, cross-country skiing, rollerblading, rowing, or swimming. • Progression: inactive people should start gradually, using light to moderate intensity exercise for short periods of time (even < 10 min), with training sessions spread throughout the week.	

Abbreviations: FITT—frequency, intensity, time-duration, type of exercise; HIIT—High-intensity interval training; VO_2—peak oxygen uptake; SBP—systolic blood pressure; DBP—diastolic blood pressure; ECG—electrocardiogram; 1RM—One-repetition maximum; HF—Heart failure; HT—Heart transplantation; VT1—first ventilatory threshold; VT2—second ventilatory threshold; MET—metabolic equivalents.

There is a consensus in international recommendations on the frequency of resistance exercise in a cardiac patient's exercise program. Resistance training should be performed 2–3 days per week, on non-consecutive days, at a frequency of 1RM. The Portuguese Society of Cardiology emphasizes that resistance exercise should be introduced in rehabilitation only from phase II of the process, i.e., after stabilization of the condition and after discharge from the ward. Depending on the source, aerobic endurance exercise should be performed 3–6 times a week, or even daily if there are no medical contraindications and the patient responds well to the exercise. Endurance exercise can last from 5–20 min to 60 min. Aerobic training should be modified by checking the parameters of fatigue, response to exercise, increasing or decreasing the intensity and duration. French recommendations suggest that training should be divided into three elements: warm-up, main part, and recovery, which will help the patient to adapt to the exercise. When recommending high-intensity interval training, the organizations emphasize the need to constantly monitor the patient's health and rule out contraindications to intense exercise. The Polish recommendation is to start training with 10 s to 4 min of moderate or high intensity, then progress to 1–3 min of low or moderate intensity. This particular form of activity should be decided on a patient-by-patient basis by a medical doctor. American organizations do not recommend extreme high-frequency exercise for heart patients. Exercise intensities should be increased cautiously and gradually, taking into account the patient's individual capabilities and health status. Given that physical training represents a core aspect of CR, it is essential to gain a comprehensive understanding of the function of mitochondrial respiration during exercise in patients with cardiovascular disease.

4. Mitochondria Overview in Cardiology and Cardiac Rehabilitation (CR)

In the cardiovascular system, mitochondria are essential for maintaining myocardial bioenergetics, supporting continuous ATP production required for cardiac contraction and vascular function. Impaired mitochondrial function is linked to heart failure, ischemic injury, and endothelial dysfunction, contributing to vascular aging and atherosclerosis [20–22]. Beyond their role in disease, mitochondria are critical for endurance performance, as their content, efficiency, and respiratory capacity correlate with maximal oxygen uptake (VO_2 max), time-trial performance, and lactate threshold [23,24]. Cardiomyocytes are highly dependent on mitochondrial oxidative phosphorylation for ATP generation. Mitochondria provide cardiomyocytes with a continuous energy supply that is essential for their dependence on repetitive calcium (Ca^{2+})-dependent contractile activity. Consequently, reduced bioenergetic efficiency of the mitochondrial network can directly impair cardiac contraction. When the mitochondrial network is damaged, the delicate balance of Ca^{2+} homeostasis and inflammatory regulation is disrupted, leading to alterations in normal cardiac function, including impaired systolic and diastolic function, arrhythmias, arterial stenosis, and other pathological manifestations [25]. Mitochondria are double-membrane organelles responsible for cellular energy production through oxidative phosphorylation (OXPHOS). They vary in size (0.1–5.0 μm in diameter) and form a highly interconnected reticular network, facilitating efficient energy distribution and adaptation to fluctuating metabolic demands [26]. These organelles contain their own mitochondrial DNA (mtDNA), encoding 37 genes, including 13 essential polypeptides of the electron transport chain (ETC). However, the majority of mitochondrial proteins (approximately 1100) are nuclear-encoded and imported into the mitochondria through specialized translocases [27].

4.1. Mitochondria Biogenesis

The primary regulator of this process is peroxisome proliferator-activated receptor gamma coactivator-1α (PGC-1α), which serves as a master transcriptional coactivator governing mitochondrial energy metabolism. Its activation in response to exercise is orchestrated through multiple signaling pathways, including AMP-activated protein kinase (AMPK) and sirtuin deacetylase 1 (SIRT1), both of which are sensitive to cellular energy status, as reflected by ATP and NAD^+ availability [28]. During exercise, recruitment of muscle myofibril motor units generates an action potential that induces the release of Ca^{2+} ions by the sarcoplasmic reticulum. Subsequently, the increase in cytoplasmic Ca^{2+} stimulates ATP synthesis and the production of ROS in mitochondria. This process promotes the translocation of PGC-1α, which increases gene transcription by interacting with transcription factors and accessory proteins on DNA promoters and regulates the expression of NuGEMPs (nuclear genes encoding mitochondrial proteins). Newly synthesized nuclear-derived proteins are then transported into mitochondria by transferases located in the outer and inner mitochondrial membrane, leading to the activation of the mitochondrial misfolded protein response and mitochondrial biogenesis, promoting their protection and repair [29]. Increased energy consumption during exercise leads also to an elevated AMP and ADP against ATP, triggering AMPK activation via phosphorylation of its catalytic α-subunit (Thr172) by liver kinase B1 (LKB1) and Ca^{2+}/calmodulin-dependent protein kinase β (CaMKKβ) [30]. Activated AMPK directly phosphorylates PGC-1α, enhancing its transcriptional activity and stability, while also increasing its expression through PPARGC1A gene induction [31]. Simultaneously, AMPK enhances SIRT1 activity by increasing cellular NAD+ levels, resulting in the deacetylation and modulation of the activity of downstream SIRT1 targets including PGC-1α and the forkhead box O1 (FOXO1) and O3 (FOXO3a) transcription factors [32]. This post-translational modification enhances PGC-1α's functional capacity, strengthening its interaction with transcription factors NRF 1 and 2 (nuclear respiratory factor 1 and 2) and NFE2L2 (nuclear factor erythroid 2-related factor 2), which orchestrate the transcription of genes critical for mitochondrial biogenesis [33]. NRF1 regulates the expression of genes encoding components of the respiratory chain [cytochrome C oxidase subunit IV (COXIV)], mitochondrial transcription factors [transcription factor A mitochondrial (TFAM), transcription factor B1 mitochondrial (TFB1M), and transcription factor B2 mitochondrial (TFB2M)], and proteins engaged in mitochondrial trans-membrane transport [translocase of the inner membrane (TIM) and translocase of the outer membrane (TOM) complexes] [34–36], while NFE2L2 regulates mitochondrial biogenesis and protects against oxidative stress by (1) enhancing NRF1 expression, promoting mitochondrial gene transcription for OXPHOS and protein import, and (2) directly activating redox-related genes, such as heme oxyenase-1 (HO-1) and superoxide dismutase 1 (SOD1) [37,38].

4.2. Mitochondria Fusion and Fission

In response to exercise or other endogenous and exogenous stimuli, mitochondria dynamically alter their morphology and function through biogenesis, mitophagy, fission, and fusion. Each of these processes is tightly regulated by specific molecular mechanisms, ensuring mitochondrial adaptability and homeostasis [39]. These processes are tightly regulated by a set of GTPase proteins, including mitofusin 1 (Mfn1), mitofusin 2 (Mfn2), optic atrophy 1 (OPA1), and fission 1 (Fis1), dynamin-related protein 1 (Drp1). Fusion, mediated by Mfn1, Mfn2, and OPA1, promotes the merging of mitochondria, allowing for content mixing (enabling the exchange of mtDNA, proteins, and metabolites), efficient ATP production, and OXPHOS optimization. In contrast, fission, regulated by Drp1 and Fis1, facilitates the removal of damaged mitochondria via mitophagy, redistribution of mitochondria during cell division, and metabolic adaptation to stress [40]. One of the crucial proteins in fission is also PTEN-induced kinase 1 (PINK1), which, by accumulating on the outer mitochondrial membrane in response to mitochondrial damage and phosphorylates Drp1 (Ser616), promotes mitochondrial division and interacts with Fis1 to stabilize this process [41]. The balance between these opposing processes is essential for mitochondrial homeostasis [42].

4.3. Mitophagy

Mitophagy is a selective autophagic process that removes damaged or dysfunctional mitochondria, ensuring mitochondrial quality control and cellular homeostasis. It is initiated when a loss of mitochondrial membrane potential ($\Delta\Psi m$) leads to PINK1 accumulation on the outer mitochondrial membrane, triggering the recruitment and activation of Parkin, an E3 ubiquitin ligase. Parkin ubiquitinates mitochondrial proteins such as Mfn1/Mfn2, marking the organelle for degradation. Ubiquitinated mitochondria are then recognized by autophagy adaptors, such as p62/SQSTM1 (sequestosome 1), nuclear dot protein 52kDA (NDP52), and optineurin (OPTN), leading to the formation of an autophagosome. The autophagosome then fuses with a lysosome, forming an autolysosome, where mitochondrial components are degraded and recycled [43].

4.4. Effects of Physical Exercise on Mitochondria Biogenesis and Functionality in Cardiological Patients

Cardiovascular diseases (CVDs) remain the leading cause of morbidity and mortality worldwide. CVDs encompass a broad spectrum of conditions characterized by impaired cardiac and vascular function, often driven by metabolic dysregulation, oxidative stress, and chronic inflammation, which are closely linked to mitochondrial dysfunction [44]. These pathophysiological processes contribute to progressive tissue damage, including apoptosis, fibrosis, and remodeling of myocardium and vasculature, which ultimately compromise cardiovascular performance. Exercise training helps counteract these effects by reducing cell death, inflammation, and fibrosis of myocardium, while promoting vascular regeneration through improved mitochondrial redox balance [45]. Regular physical activity and exercise play a crucial role in postponing the development of CVDs. One key factor in the progression of CVDs is the disruption of mitochondrial homeostasis. Exercise training effectively slows both the onset and advancement of these diseases by restoring mitochondrial balance. This involves enhancing mitochondrial biogenesis, promoting fusion while reducing fission, stimulating mitophagy, and preserving mitochondrial structure and function [46]. These conditions are also characterized by a significant regulation of mitochondria-derived intracellular signaling, including reactive oxygen species (ROS) and Ca^{2+} homeostasis [47].

The progressive decline in mitochondrial function in CVDs is linked to respiratory chain alterations and impaired ATP synthesis, leading to cardiomyocyte damage and death. This occurs through apoptosis, triggered by cytochrome c release, or necrosis, induced by mitochondrial permeability transition pore (PTP) opening [48]. Inhibiting mPTP is widely recognized as a strategy to reduce cardiomyocyte loss, which contributes to conditions such as myocardial ischemia-reperfusion injury, various cardiomyopathies, and cardiotoxicity [49]. While large, randomized studies on mitochondrial-targeted therapies in CVDs are lacking, numerous preclinical studies highlight mitochondria as a promising therapeutic target. Given their crucial role in energy production and oxidative stress regulation, especially in non-dividing, high-energy-demand cells like cardiomyocytes, maintaining mitochondrial integrity is essential. Coordinating quality control mechanisms including mitochondrial biogenesis, dynamics, and mitophagy, may help prevent mitochondrial dysfunction and slow CVD progression [50–52]. All necessary influences of exercise on mitochondrial biogenesis and function in CVD patients are present on Figure 2.

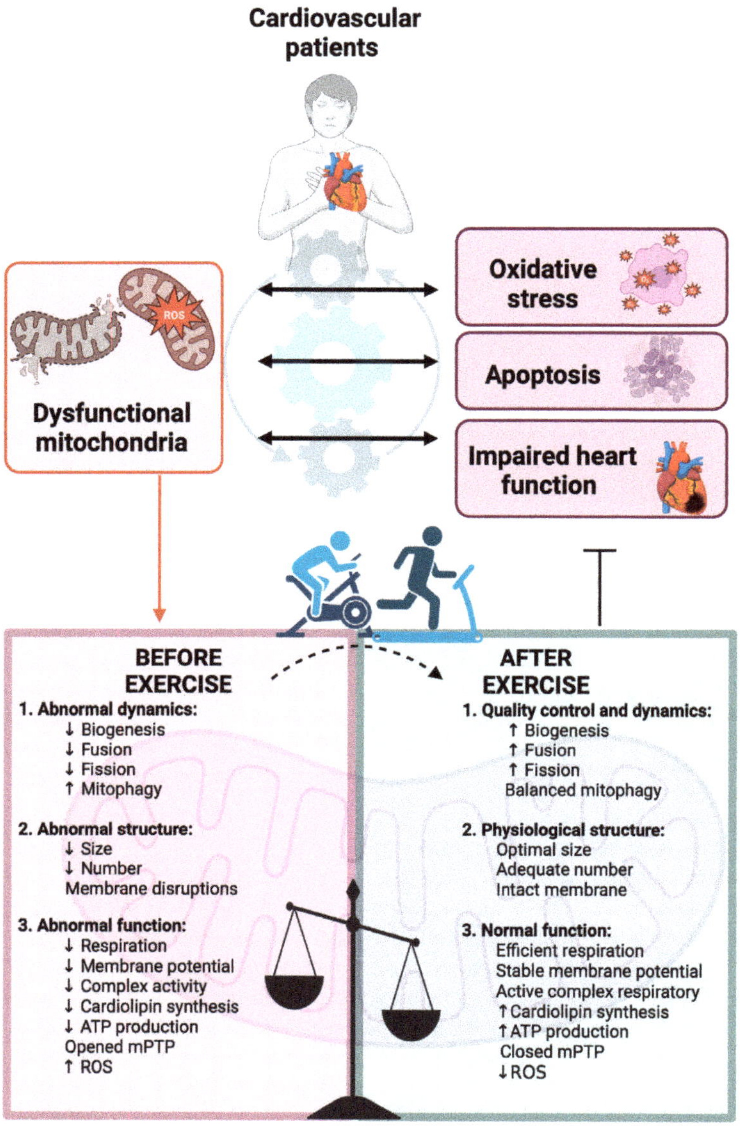

Figure 2. Exercise-induced mitochondrial restoration in cardiovascular (CVD) patients. The role of mitochondrial dysfunction in CVD progression and the beneficial effects of exercise. Damaged mitochondria contribute to oxidative stress, apoptosis, and impaired cardiac function. Regular physical activity restores mitochondrial biogenesis, dynamics, structure, and function, reducing cellular stress and supporting heart performance. Abbreviations: ATP—adenosine triphosphate; mPTP—mitochondrial permeability transition pore; ROS—reactive oxygen species. Created in BioRender. Dziedzic, A. (2025), https://BioRender.com/hte5bak (accessed on 29 May 2025).

Mitochondrial biogenesis and functional adaptation to exercise are key determinants of aerobic capacity and cardiovascular resilience. Long-term activation of AMPK through regular physical exercise induces important metabolic changes, such as greater mitochondrial sensitivity and optimization of energy metabolism [53]. Physical exercise is a key factor that stimulates mitochondrial biogenesis, which is fundamental in efficient cardiomyocyte metabolism and optimizing cardiac muscle function [54–56]. Exercise increases the AMP:ATP ratio, leading to allosteric activation of AMPK, which triggers multiple signaling pathways, including those involved in mitochondrial biogenesis. Regular exercise activates AMPK, enhancing mitochondrial fission and fusion. Campos et al.'s in vivo study demonstrated that a single 4-h swim triggered mitochondrial fragmentation, followed by fusion during recovery, while long-term swimming delayed mitochondrial fragmentation [57]. Mice lacking AMPK $\beta1/\beta2$ isoforms in skeletal muscle show severe physical inactivity and reduced treadmill endurance, linked to lower mitochondrial content [58]. Similarly, AMPK$\alpha1\alpha2$ knockout mice exhibit weakened exercise capacity, decreased maximal force production, and fatigue resistance, primarily due to complex I dysfunction [59]. Ju et al. report that eight weeks of regular swimming improved mitochondrial biogenesis in skeletal muscle of mice by increasing the expression of PGC-1α and key markers of mitochondrial biogenesis, such as succinate dehydrogenase and cytochrome c oxidase-IV [60]. Likewise, an 8-week moderate-intensity treadmill training program reduced excessive mitochondrial fission and inflammation in the soleus muscle of diabetic rats [61]. Exercise modulates exerkines (musclin, follistatin, and myonectin), which enhance metabolism, inflammation control, and cardiovascular function, helping to reduce cardiac fibrosis, remodeling, and dysfunction after ischemia [62]. Four weeks of treadmill training improved mitochondrial integrity and biogenesis, reducing myocardial damage via SIRT1/PGC-1α/PI3K/Akt activation [63]. In MI mice, eight weeks of swimming (15 min/day) lowered two key mitohphagy markers—microtubule-associated protein 1 light chain 3-II (LC3-II) and p62 levels, while increasing PINK/Parkin expression, enhancing mitophagy. Moderate training elevated SIRT3 levels, reducing ROS, apoptosis, and fibrosis under hypoxic conditions [64].

The few existing human studies align with findings from in vivo research, confirming the same direction of mitochondrial adaptations to exercise. Mendham et al. showed that a 12-week combined aerobic and endurance training program increased the levels of specific intermediate lipids in skeletal muscle, including cardiolipin, phosphatidylcholine, and phosphatidylethanolamine, and enhanced the function of mitochondrial complexes I–V. As a result, respiratory capacity and mitochondrial biogenesis were significantly improved [65]. Endurance training increases mitochondrial volume by 40–50%, leads to higher mitochondrial protein content, improving β-oxidation, and electron transport chain functioning [65]. Mitokines, such as fibroblast growth factor 21 (FGF21) and growth differentiation factor 15 (GDF15), are signaling molecules that mediate mitochondrial communication and stress adaptation. Exercise helps maintain mitochondrial protein homeostasis by regulating mitokine expression. An 8-week endurance training program increased FGF21 levels, exercise capacity, and muscle fiber distribution, while GDF15, a stress-responsive myokine and cardiokine, was elevated during intensive exercise, highlighting its role in exercise-induced adaptations [66]. Porter et al. demonstrated that 12 weeks of resistance exercise training led to both qualitative and quantitative enhancements in skeletal muscle mitochondrial respiration, despite only modest changes in mitochondrial protein content and gene expression. These findings suggest that resistance training effectively improves mitochondrial respiratory capacity and intrinsic function, highlighting its role in optimizing skeletal muscle bioenergetics [23]. The multifaceted impact of exercise on mitochondrial health through molecular signaling pathways that enhance biogenesis, protein synthesis, dynamics, mitophagy, and oxidative phosphorylation are presented on Figure 3.

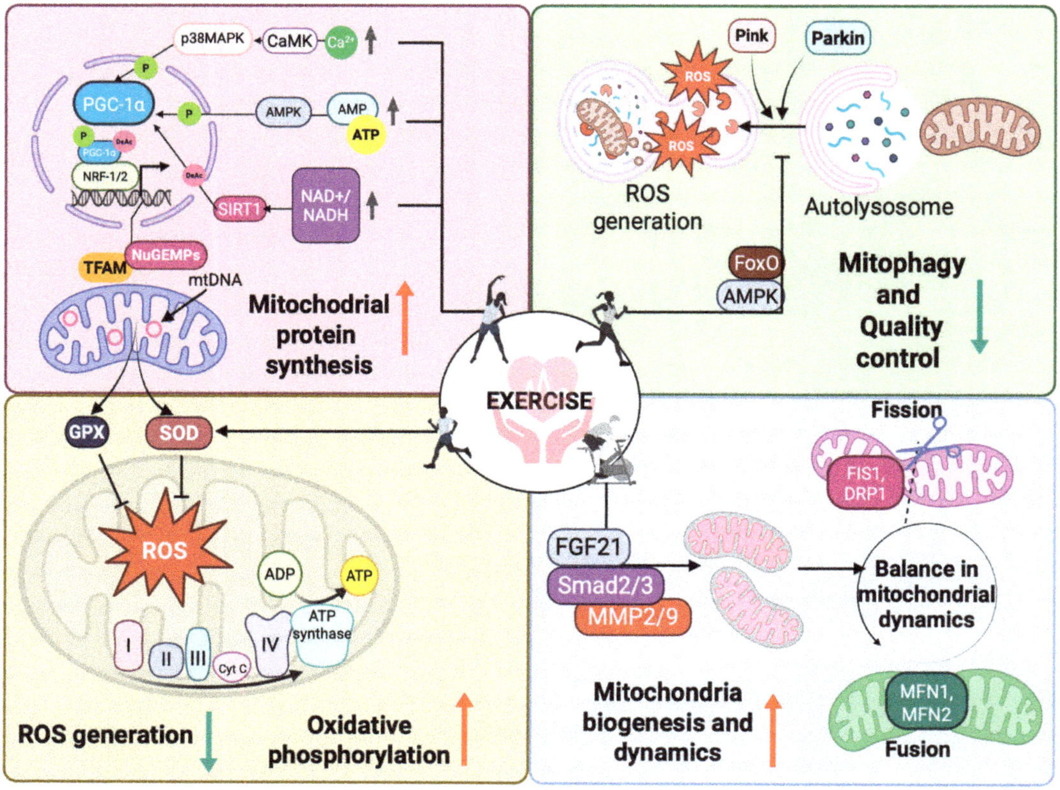

Figure 3. Molecular mechanisms and signaling pathways underlying exercise-induced mitochondrial adaptations. In the upper left panel, exercise activates key regulators such as AMPK, CaMK, and p38MAPK, leading to the upregulation of PGC-1α and downstream transcription factors (NRF-1/2, TFAM), thereby promoting mitochondrial protein synthesis and mtDNA transcription. SIRT1 activation via NAD^+ also supports this process. In the lower left panel, enhanced antioxidant defenses (e.g., SOD, GPX) and more efficient electron transport chain activity reduce reactive oxygen species (ROS) generation and improve oxidative phosphorylation, leading to increased ATP production. The upper right panel depicts exercise-induced activation of mitophagy and mitochondrial quality control via the Pink1/Parkin pathway. Exercise upregulates AMPK and FoxO signaling, promoting the removal of damaged mitochondria through autophagosome formation and lysosomal degradation. The lower right panel shows improvements in mitochondrial biogenesis and dynamics. Exercise promotes the expression of FGF21 and activation of Smad2/3 and MMP2/9 pathways, restoring the balance between mitochondrial fission (FIS1, DRP1) and fusion (MFN1, MFN2), which is essential for maintaining mitochondrial integrity and function. Abbreviations: AMPK—AMP-activated protein kinase; ATP—adenosine triphosphate; CaMK—calcium/calmodulin-dependent protein kinase; DRP1—dynamin-related protein 1; FGF21—fibroblast growth factor 21; FIS1—fission 1 protein; FoxO—forkhead box O; GPX—glutathione peroxidase; MFN1—mitofusin 1; MFN2—mitofusin 2; MMP2—matrix metalloproteinase 2; MMP9—matrix metalloproteinase 9; mtDNA—mitochondrial DNA; NAD+—nicotinamide adenine dinucleotide; NRF-1/2—nuclear respiratory factor 1 and 2; NuGEMPs—nuclear genome-encoded mitochondrial proteins; PGC-1α—peroxisome proliferator-activated receptor gamma coactivator 1-alpha; Pink1—PTEN-induced kinase 1; Parkin—E3 ubiquitin ligase Parkin; ROS—reactive oxygen species; SIRT1—sirtuin 1; Smad2/3—mothers against decapentaplegic homolog 2 and 3; SOD—superoxide dismutase; TFAM—mitochondrial transcription factor A. Created in BioRender. Dziedzic, A. (2025), https://BioRender.com/bhes4bs (accessed on 29 May 2025).

4.5. Non-Invasive Potential Methods for Assessing Mitochondrial Adaptation

Recent studies highlight the importance of assessing exercise effectiveness by identifying biomarkers that reflect functional status and potential mitochondrial adaptations in patients. Various "omics" approaches, such as transcriptomics and proteomics, offer a comprehensive insight into the genes and proteins involved in mitochondrial biogenesis, revealing their dynamic changes in response to high-intensity exercise. One of the newest approaches to assessing this condition is the measurement of mitochondrial microRNAs (mitomiRs) expression [67,68]. Research underlines the crucial role of mitomiRs in regulating biological adaptations of cardiovascular system to physical activity, such as cardiac muscle growth, mitochondrial biogenesis, vascular development, and metabolic regulation [69]. The exploration of mitomiRs as biomarkers of mitochondrial adaptation is still in its early stages, with only a handful of studies available. However, this emerging field holds immense potential, offering a promising avenue for understanding how mitochondria respond to physiological stress and exercise. Research by Carrer et al. has shown that miR-378 plays a key role in regulating mitochondrial energy production by modulating the expression of PGC1-β, at which elevated levels are commonly observed as a physiological response to endurance exercise [70]. Furthermore, miR-494 plays a pivotal role in mitochondrial biogenesis within skeletal muscle [71,72], while also acting as a negative regulator of SIRT3, a key enzyme that fine-tunes mitochondrial energy metabolism in response to exercise and nutritional signals [72,73]. This dual function positions miR-494 as a critical player in balancing mitochondrial adaptation and metabolic flexibility.

Another method worth noting in this field is a single-cell RNA sequencing (scRNA-seq). This technology allows researchers to examine how different cell populations within tissues, such as skeletal muscle or cardiac tissue, respond to physical activity at the transcriptional level. A study utilizing scRNA-seq to explored exercise-induced cardiac adaptations by analyzing mitochondrial gene expression related to fission–fusion balance in heart tissues. By comparing exercised mouse hearts with bulk RNA-seq data, researchers found that exercise modulates mitochondrial fusion and fission processes, which are critical for cardiac adaptation. Specific mitochondrial gene clusters exhibited increased expression post-exercise, suggesting enhanced mitochondrial biogenesis and metabolic flexibility. The study highlighted that maintaining a dynamic balance between mitochondrial fusion and fission is essential for cardiovascular health and the adaptive responses to exercise [74].

Mitochondrial respiration is a fundamental process in cellular metabolism, driving energy conversion through enzymatically regulated reactions that transform substrate-derived energy into ATP. The Seahorse analyzer enables real-time measurement of oxygen consumption in living cells, providing valuable insights into mitochondrial function. This technology allows for the assessment of four key parameters of mitochondrial respiration: basal respiration, ATP-linked respiration, maximal respiration, and proton leak, offering a comprehensive evaluation of mitochondrial efficiency and bioenergetic health. A study by Pribil Pardun et al. investigated mitochondrial adaptation in C2C12 myotubes using electrical pulse stimulation as a model for exercise training. Their findings suggest that mitochondrial bioenergetic profiles improve in response to chronic stimulation, mimicking endurance exercise adaptations [75]. Another promising technique is imaging with MitoTimer, a fluorescent probe distinguishing newly formed mitochondria (green fluorescence) from older ones (red fluorescence) [76], which confirmed enhanced mitochondrial biogenesis in exercised mice, as indicated by a shift toward green fluorescence. In contrast, a high-fat diet promotes red fluorescence, suggesting reduced biogenesis, an effect counteracted by exercise [77].

Looking ahead, future research should prioritize longitudinal human studies directly investigating mitochondrial adaptations to structured CR programs. Such studies are critical to validate preclinical findings and establish clinically relevant mechanisms underlying exercise-induced cardioprotection. In parallel, efforts should focus on the identification and validation of circulating biomarkers, including mitomiRs or other exerkines (signaling molecules released into circulation during and after physical exercise, contributing to systemic adaptations) to monitor mitochondrial function and responsiveness to exercise. These molecular indicators could support personalized exercise prescriptions, stratify patients by responsiveness, and enhance the translational impact of mitochondrial-targeted therapies in cardiovascular care.

5. Limitations

The article has some limitations. It discusses CR in the context of European and American populations, omitting data from Asia, Africa, and other regions of the world. A study by Supervia et al. characterizing CR programs around the world indicates the program's availability in Africa. However, only eight countries in Africa have CR programs available for patients: Algeria, Benin, Kenya, Mauritius, Nigeria, South Africa, Tanzania, and Uganda. In Asian regions, the authors collected data from the Eastern Mediterranean (EMR), South-East Asia (SEAR), and the Western Pacific (WPR). CR programs were available in 12 EMR countries, including Afghanistan, Bahrain, Iran, Kuwait, Pakistan, Lebanon, Qatar, and Saudi Arabia), 6 SEAR countries (Bangladesh, India, Indonesia, Nepal, Sri Lanka, and Thailand), and 11 Western Pacific countries (Brunei Darussalam, China, Malaysia, Japan, the Philippines, Mongolia, Singapore, South Korea, and Taiwan). The African region shows much lower CR availability compared to the EMR, SEAR, and WPR [78]. CR availability by continent is 17% in Africa [79]. There is a lack of guidance on how to implement CR programs in low-resource settings, particularly in Africa [79]. The available Asian–Pacific recommendations offer regional insights into the objectives and prevalence of CR programs [80]. Despite the greater implementation of CR programs in this region, there is a lack of unified recommendations with detailed information on rehabilitation programs, medical personnel, and specific cardiological diseases. These data were not included in the review due to the lack of detailed and standardized information on CR programs in the African, EMR, SEAR, and WPR. Future studies analyzing CR programs should focus on areas with limited financial resources and high continental latitude, which affect access to CR disparities. Future analyses should compare CR programs in the following regions: Europe, America, Africa, Asia, and Australia.

Another limitation of this study is that most of the evidence presented in this section originates from preclinical animal models. While these studies have significantly advanced our understanding of mitochondrial adaptations to exercise, they present several limitations in terms of clinical translation. First, species-specific differences in cardiac metabolism, mitochondrial biogenesis rates, and redox signaling pathways mean that mechanisms observed in rodents may not fully replicate those in humans. Additionally, the exercise protocols used in animal studies (e.g., forced treadmill or swimming) often differ in intensity, duration, and physiological relevance compared to human rehabilitation programs. Moreover, animal models typically lack comorbidities (such as diabetes, hypertension, or medication use) commonly present in cardiovascular patients, limiting the generalizability of findings. Despite strong evidence supporting the crucial role of exercise in mitochondrial function, particularly in cardiovascular health, research remains largely limited to in vivo studies, with a notable lack of human trials. This gap poses a challenge to translating molecular insights into evidence-based clinical recommendations. To address this, future research should prioritize longitudinal human studies that integrate molecular, physiological, and clinical outcomes to validate the therapeutic potential of targeting mitochondrial pathways in CR.

6. Conclusions and Future Perspectives

Physical activity is a cornerstone of CR and a critical element of evidence-based secondary prevention strategies recommended by leading cardiology societies. Beyond its well-established clinical benefits, regular exercise induces profound mitochondrial adaptations, including enhanced biogenesis, improved oxidative phosphorylation efficiency, and greater resilience to oxidative stress. These cellular-level changes contribute to improved cardiac function and vascular health by promoting endothelial function, facilitating angiogenesis, and reducing systemic inflammation. Importantly, these biological mechanisms align with clinical guidelines that advocate for structured exercise interventions, such as aerobic and resistance training, tailored to individual patient profiles. These interventions have been shown to reduce the incidence of recurrent cardiovascular events, lower all-cause mortality, and improve quality of life in patients with coronary artery disease, heart failure, and other cardiovascular conditions. Incorporating mitochondrial health as a therapeutic target within these guidelines could further optimize rehabilitation outcomes. Future research should aim to refine exercise prescriptions based on molecular markers of mitochondrial function and explore synergistic strategies combining exercise with pharmacological agents that support mitochondrial integrity. In this context, physical activity not only enhances cellular resilience but also operationalizes the principles of precision medicine in cardiovascular care.

Author Contributions: Conceptualization, A.D., D.S. and E.M.; methodology, K.M. and A.D.; software, K.M.; validation, D.S., E.M., K.M. and A.D.; formal analysis, E.M.; investigation, K.M., A.D., P.N. (Patrycja Nowak) and P.N. (Piotr Niebrzydowski); resources, P.N. (Patrycja Nowak) and P.N. (Piotr Niebrzydowski); data curation, K.M. and A.D.; writing—original draft preparation, A.D., K.M., P.N. (Patrycja Nowak), D.S. and E.M.; writing—review and editing, A.D., E.M. and D.S.; visualization, K.M. and A.D.; supervision, E.M.; project administration, E.M.; funding acquisition, E.M. All authors have read and agreed to the published version of the manuscript.

Funding: This research received no external funding.

Institutional Review Board Statement: Not applicable.

Informed Consent Statement: Not applicable.

Conflicts of Interest: The authors declare no conflicts of interest.

References

1. Ambrosetti, M.; Abreu, A.; Corrà, U.; Davos, C.H.; Hansen, D.; Frederix, I.; Iliou, M.C.; Pedretti, R.F.; Schmid, J.-P.; Vigorito, C. Secondary prevention through comprehensive cardiovascular rehabilitation: From knowledge to implementation. 2020 update. A position paper from the Secondary Prevention and Rehabilitation Section of the European Association of Preventive Cardiology. *Eur. J. Prev. Cardiol.* **2021**, *28*, 460–495. [CrossRef] [PubMed]
2. Jegier, A.; Szalewska, D.; Mawlichanów, A.; Bednarczyk, T.; Eysymontt, Z.; Gałaszek, M.; Mamcarz, A.; Mierzyńska, A.; Piotrowicz, E.; Piotrowicz, R. Comprehensive cardiac rehabilitation as the keystone in the secondary prevention of cardiovascular disease. *Pol. Heart J.* **2021**, *79*, 901–916. [CrossRef] [PubMed]
3. Cowie, A.; Buckley, J.; Doherty, P.; Furze, G.; Hayward, J.; Hinton, S.; Jones, J.; Speck, L.; Dalal, H.; Mills, J. Standards and core components for cardiovascular disease prevention and rehabilitation. *Heart* **2019**, *105*, 510–515. [CrossRef] [PubMed]
4. Lim, A.Y.; Chen, Y.-C.; Hsu, C.-C.; Fu, T.-C.; Wang, J.-S. The effects of exercise training on mitochondrial function in cardiovascular diseases: A systematic review and meta-analysis. *Int. J. Mol. Sci.* **2022**, *23*, 12559. [CrossRef]
5. Zeng, Z.; Yuan, Q.; Zu, X.; Liu, J. Insights into the role of mitochondria in vascular calcification. *Front. Cardiovasc. Med.* **2022**, *9*, 879752. [CrossRef]
6. Dalal, J.; Low, L.-P.; Van Phuoc, D.; Abdul Rahman, A.R.; Reyes, E.; Ann Soenarta, A.; Tomlinson, B. The use of medications in the secondary prevention of coronary artery disease in the Asian region. *Curr. Med. Res. Opin.* **2015**, *31*, 423–433. [CrossRef]
7. Pavy, B.; Iliou, M.-C.; Vergès-Patois, B.; Brion, R.; Monpère, C.; Carré, F.; Aeberhard, P.; Argouach, C.; Borgne, A.; Consoli, S. French Society of Cardiology guidelines for cardiac rehabilitation in adults. *Arch. Cardiovasc. Dis.* **2012**, *105*, 309–328. [CrossRef]

8. Mamataz, T.; Uddin, J.; Alam, S.I.; Taylor, R.S.; Pakosh, M.; Grace, S.L. Effects of cardiac rehabilitation in low- and middle-income countries: A systematic review and meta-analysis of randomised controlled trials. *Prog. Cardiovasc. Dis.* **2022**, *70*, 119–174. [CrossRef]
9. Dibben, G.O.; Faulkner, J.; Oldridge, N.; Rees, K.; Thompson, D.R.; Zwisler, A.-D.; Taylor, R.S. Exercise-based cardiac rehabilitation for coronary heart disease: A meta-analysis. *Eur. Heart J.* **2023**, *44*, 452–469. [CrossRef]
10. Bigot, M.; Guy, J.M.; Monpere, C.; Cohen-Solal, A.; Pavy, B.; Iliou, M.C.; Bosser, G.; Corone, S.; Douard, H.; Farrokhi, T. Cardiac rehabilitation recommendations of the Group Exercise Rehabilitation Sports–Prevention (GERS-P) of the French Society of Cardiology: 2023 update. *Arch. Cardiovasc. Dis.* **2024**, *117*, 521–541. [CrossRef]
11. Brown, T.M.; Pack, Q.R.; Aberegg, E.; Brewer, L.C.; Ford, Y.R.; Forman, D.E.; Gathright, E.C.; Khadanga, S.; Ozemek, C.; Thomas, R.J. Core components of cardiac rehabilitation programs: 2024 update: A scientific statement from the American Heart Association and the American Association of Cardiovascular and Pulmonary Rehabilitation. *Circulation* **2024**, *150*, e328–e347. [CrossRef] [PubMed]
12. Abreu, A.; Mendes, M.; Dores, H.; Silveira, C.; Fontes, P.; Teixeira, M.; Santa Clara, H.; Morais, J. Mandatory criteria for cardiac rehabilitation programs: 2018 guidelines from the Portuguese Society of Cardiology. *Rev. Port. Cardiol.* **2018**, *37*, 363–373. [CrossRef] [PubMed]
13. Piepoli, M.F.; Hoes, A.W.; Agewall, S.; Albus, C.; Brotons, C.; Catapano, A.L.; Cooney, M.-T.; Corrà, U.; Cosyns, B.; Deaton, C. 2016 European Guidelines on cardiovascular disease prevention in clinical practice. *Pol. Heart J.* **2016**, *74*, 821–936. [CrossRef] [PubMed]
14. Zielińska-Nowak, E.; Cichon, N.; Saluk-Bijak, J.; Bijak, M.; Miller, E. Nutritional supplements and neuroprotective diets and their potential clinical significance in post-stroke rehabilitation. *Nutrients* **2021**, *13*, 2704. [CrossRef] [PubMed]
15. Lavie, C.J.; Milani, R.V. Cardiac rehabilitation and exercise training in secondary coronary heart disease prevention. *Prog. Cardiovasc. Dis.* **2011**, *53*, 397–403. [CrossRef]
16. Kirkman, D.L.; Lee, D.-c.; Carbone, S. Resistance exercise for cardiac rehabilitation. *Prog. Cardiovasc. Dis.* **2022**, *70*, 66–72. [CrossRef]
17. Xanthos, P.D.; Gordon, B.A.; Kingsley, M.I. Implementing resistance training in the rehabilitation of coronary heart disease: A systematic review and meta-analysis. *Int. J. Cardiol.* **2017**, *230*, 493–508. [CrossRef]
18. Jelleyman, C.; Yates, T.; O'Donovan, G.; Gray, L.J.; King, J.A.; Khunti, K.; Davies, M.J. The effects of high-intensity interval training on glucose regulation and insulin resistance: A meta-analysis. *Obes. Rev.* **2015**, *16*, 942–961. [CrossRef]
19. Ruivo, J.; Moholdt, T.; Abreu, A. Overview of Cardiac Rehabilitation following post-acute myocardial infarction in European Society of Cardiology member countries. *Eur. J. Prev. Cardiol.* **2023**, *30*, 758–768. [CrossRef]
20. Brown, D.A.; Perry, J.B.; Allen, M.E.; Sabbah, H.N.; Stauffer, B.L.; Shaikh, S.R.; Cleland, J.G.; Colucci, W.S.; Butler, J.; Voors, A.A. Mitochondrial function as a therapeutic target in heart failure. *Nat. Rev. Cardiol.* **2017**, *14*, 238–250. [CrossRef]
21. Qu, K.; Yan, F.; Qin, X.; Zhang, K.; He, W.; Dong, M.; Wu, G. Mitochondrial dysfunction in vascular endothelial cells and its role in atherosclerosis. *Front. Physiol.* **2022**, *13*, 1084604. [CrossRef] [PubMed]
22. Ham, P.B., III; Raju, R. Mitochondrial function in hypoxic ischemic injury and influence of aging. *Prog. Neurobiol.* **2017**, *157*, 92–116. [CrossRef] [PubMed]
23. Porter, C.; Reidy, P.T.; Bhattarai, N.; Sidossis, L.S.; Rasmussen, B.B. Resistance exercise training alters mitochondrial function in human skeletal muscle. *Med. Sci. Sports Exerc.* **2015**, *47*, 1922–1931. [CrossRef] [PubMed]
24. Powers, S.K.; Radak, Z.; Ji, L.L.; Jackson, M. Reactive oxygen species promote endurance exercise-induced adaptations in skeletal muscles. *J. Sport Health Sci.* **2024**, *13*, 780–792. [CrossRef]
25. Huang, Y.; Zhou, B. Mitochondrial dysfunction in cardiac diseases and therapeutic strategies. *Biomedicines* **2023**, *11*, 1500. [CrossRef]
26. Yan, W.; Diao, S.; Fan, Z. The role and mechanism of mitochondrial functions and energy metabolism in the function regulation of the mesenchymal stem cells. *Stem Cell Res. Ther.* **2021**, *12*, 140. [CrossRef]
27. Lax, N.Z.; Turnbull, D.M.; Reeve, A.K. Mitochondrial mutations: Newly discovered players in neuronal degeneration. *Neurosci.* **2011**, *17*, 645–658. [CrossRef]
28. Abu Shelbayeh, O.; Arroum, T.; Morris, S.; Busch, K.B. PGC-1α is a master regulator of mitochondrial lifecycle and ROS stress response. *Antioxidants* **2023**, *12*, 1075. [CrossRef]
29. Scarpulla, R.C.; Vega, R.B.; Kelly, D.P. Transcriptional integration of mitochondrial biogenesis. *Trends Endocrinol. Metab.* **2012**, *23*, 459–466. [CrossRef]
30. Willows, R.; Sanders, M.J.; Xiao, B.; Patel, B.R.; Martin, S.R.; Read, J.; Wilson, J.R.; Hubbard, J.; Gamblin, S.J.; Carling, D. Phosphorylation of AMPK by upstream kinases is required for activity in mammalian cells. *Biochem. J.* **2017**, *474*, 3059–3073. [CrossRef]
31. Irrcher, I.; Ljubicic, V.; Kirwan, A.F.; Hood, D.A. AMP-activated protein kinase-regulated activation of the PGC-1α promoter in skeletal muscle cells. *PLoS ONE* **2008**, *3*, e3614. [CrossRef] [PubMed]

32. Lee, D.; Goldberg, A.L. SIRT1 protein, by blocking the activities of transcription factors FoxO1 and FoxO3, inhibits muscle atrophy and promotes muscle growth. *J. Biol. Chem.* **2013**, *288*, 30515–30526. [CrossRef] [PubMed]
33. Fernandez-Marcos, P.J.; Auwerx, J. Regulation of PGC-1α, a nodal regulator of mitochondrial biogenesis. *Am. J. Clin. Nutr.* **2011**, *93*, 884S–890S. [CrossRef] [PubMed]
34. Yang, Z.-F.; Drumea, K.; Mott, S.; Wang, J.; Rosmarin, A.G. GABP transcription factor (nuclear respiratory factor 2) is required for mitochondrial biogenesis. *Mol. Cell. Biol.* **2014**, *34*, 3194–3201. [CrossRef]
35. Satoh, J.-i.; Kawana, N.; Yamamoto, Y. Pathway analysis of ChIP-Seq-based NRF1 target genes suggests a logical hypothesis of their involvement in the pathogenesis of neurodegenerative diseases. *Gene Regul. Syst. Biol.* **2013**, *7*, GRSB.S13204. [CrossRef]
36. Biswas, M.; Chan, J.Y. Role of Nrf1 in antioxidant response element-mediated gene expression and beyond. *Toxicol. Appl. Pharmacol.* **2010**, *244*, 16–20. [CrossRef]
37. Piantadosi, C.A.; Carraway, M.S.; Babiker, A.; Suliman, H.B. Heme oxygenase-1 regulates cardiac mitochondrial biogenesis via Nrf2-mediated transcriptional control of nuclear respiratory factor-1. *Circ. Res.* **2008**, *103*, 1232–1240. [CrossRef]
38. Malhotra, D.; Portales-Casamar, E.; Singh, A.; Srivastava, S.; Arenillas, D.; Happel, C.; Shyr, C.; Wakabayashi, N.; Kensler, T.W.; Wasserman, W.W. Global mapping of binding sites for Nrf2 identifies novel targets in cell survival response through ChIP-Seq profiling and network analysis. *Nucleic Acids Res.* **2010**, *38*, 5718–5734. [CrossRef]
39. Hughes, D.C.; Ellefsen, S.; Baar, K. Adaptations to endurance and strength training. *Cold Spring Harb. Perspect. Med.* **2018**, *8*, a029769. [CrossRef]
40. Adebayo, M.; Singh, S.; Singh, A.P.; Dasgupta, S. Mitochondrial fusion and fission: The fine-tune balance for cellular homeostasis. *FASEB J.* **2021**, *35*, e21620. [CrossRef]
41. Thomas, K.J.; Cookson, M.R. The role of PTEN-induced kinase 1 in mitochondrial dysfunction and dynamics. *Int. J. Biochem. Cell Biol.* **2009**, *41*, 2025–2035. [CrossRef] [PubMed]
42. Hall, A.; Burke, N.; Dongworth, R.; Hausenloy, D. Mitochondrial fusion and fission proteins: Novel therapeutic targets for combating cardiovascular disease. *Br. J. Pharmacol.* **2014**, *171*, 1890–1906. [CrossRef] [PubMed]
43. Geisler, S.; Holmström, K.M.; Skujat, D.; Fiesel, F.C.; Rothfuss, O.C.; Kahle, P.J.; Springer, W. PINK1/Parkin-mediated mitophagy is dependent on VDAC1 and p62/SQSTM1. *Nat. Cell Biol.* **2010**, *12*, 119–131. [CrossRef] [PubMed]
44. Di Cesare, M.; Perel, P.; Taylor, S.; Kabudula, C.; Bixby, H.; Gaziano, T.A.; McGhie, D.V.; Mwangi, J.; Pervan, B.; Narula, J. The heart of the world. *Glob. Heart* **2024**, *19*, 11. [CrossRef]
45. Zhang, C.-Y.; Li, K.-L.; Zhao, X.-X.; Zhang, Z.-Y.; Yin, A.-W.; Wang, R.-X. The Role and Underlying Mechanisms of Exercise in Heart Failure. *Rev. Cardiovasc. Med.* **2024**, *25*, 285. [CrossRef]
46. Zhang, H.; Zhang, Y.; Zhang, J.; Jia, D. Exercise Alleviates Cardiovascular Diseases by Improving Mitochondrial Homeostasis. *J. Am. Heart Assoc.* **2024**, *13*, e036555. [CrossRef]
47. Lozano, O.; Marcos, P.; Salazar-Ramirez, F.d.J.; Lázaro-Alfaro, A.F.; Sobrevia, L.; García-Rivas, G. Targeting the mitochondrial Ca^{2+} uniporter complex in cardiovascular disease. *Acta Physiol.* **2023**, *237*, e13946. [CrossRef]
48. Ikeda, Y.; Sciarretta, S.; Nagarajan, N.; Rubattu, S.; Volpe, M.; Frati, G.; Sadoshima, J. New insights into the role of mitochondrial dynamics and autophagy during oxidative stress and aging in the heart. *Oxidative Med. Cell. Longev.* **2014**, *2014*, 210934. [CrossRef]
49. Mendoza, A.; Patel, P.; Robichaux, D.; Ramirez, D.; Karch, J. Inhibition of the mPTP and lipid peroxidation is additively protective against I/R injury. *Circ. Res.* **2024**, *134*, 1292–1305. [CrossRef]
50. Yang, J.; Guo, Q.; Feng, X.; Liu, Y.; Zhou, Y. Mitochondrial dysfunction in cardiovascular diseases: Potential targets for treatment. *Front. Cell Dev. Biol.* **2022**, *10*, 841523. [CrossRef]
51. Rocca, C.; Soda, T.; De Francesco, E.M.; Fiorillo, M.; Moccia, F.; Viglietto, G.; Angelone, T.; Amodio, N. Mitochondrial dysfunction at the crossroad of cardiovascular diseases and cancer. *J. Transl. Med.* **2023**, *21*, 635. [CrossRef] [PubMed]
52. Zong, Y.; Li, H.; Liao, P.; Chen, L.; Pan, Y.; Zheng, Y.; Zhang, C.; Liu, D.; Zheng, M.; Gao, J. Mitochondrial dysfunction: Mechanisms and advances in therapy. *Signal Transduct. Target. Ther.* **2024**, *9*, 124. [CrossRef] [PubMed]
53. Plaza-Diaz, J.; Izquierdo, D.; Torres-Martos, Á.; Baig, A.T.; Aguilera, C.M.; Ruiz-Ojeda, F.J. Impact of physical activity and exercise on the epigenome in skeletal muscle and effects on systemic metabolism. *Biomedicines* **2022**, *10*, 126. [CrossRef] [PubMed]
54. MacInnis, M.J.; Zacharewicz, E.; Martin, B.J.; Haikalis, M.E.; Skelly, L.E.; Tarnopolsky, M.A.; Murphy, R.M.; Gibala, M.J. Superior mitochondrial adaptations in human skeletal muscle after interval compared to continuous single-leg cycling matched for total work. *J. Physiol.* **2017**, *595*, 2955–2968. [CrossRef]
55. Meinild Lundby, A.K.; Jacobs, R.; Gehrig, S.; De Leur, J.; Hauser, M.; Bonne, T.; Flück, D.; Dandanell, S.; Kirk, N.; Kaech, A. Exercise training increases skeletal muscle mitochondrial volume density by enlargement of existing mitochondria and not de novo biogenesis. *Acta Physiol.* **2018**, *222*, e12905. [CrossRef]
56. Serpiello, F.R.; Mckenna, M.J.; Bishop, D.J.; Aughey, R.J.; Caldow, M.K.; Cameron-Smith, D.; Stepto, N.K. Repeated sprints alter signaling related to mitochondrial biogenesis in humans. *Med. Sci. Sports Exerc.* **2012**, *44*, 827–834. [CrossRef]

57. Campos, J.C.; Marchesi Bozi, L.H.; Krum, B.; Grassmann Bechara, L.R.; Ferreira, N.D.; Arini, G.S.; Albuquerque, R.P.; Traa, A.; Ogawa, T.; van der Bliek, A.M. Exercise preserves physical fitness during aging through AMPK and mitochondrial dynamics. *Proc. Natl. Acad. Sci. USA* **2023**, *120*, e2204750120. [CrossRef]
58. O'Neill, H.M.; Maarbjerg, S.J.; Crane, J.D.; Jeppesen, J.; Jørgensen, S.B.; Schertzer, J.D.; Shyroka, O.; Kiens, B.; Van Denderen, B.J.; Tarnopolsky, M.A. AMP-activated protein kinase (AMPK) β1β2 muscle null mice reveal an essential role for AMPK in maintaining mitochondrial content and glucose uptake during exercise. *Proc. Natl. Acad. Sci. USA* **2011**, *108*, 16092–16097. [CrossRef]
59. Lantier, L.; Fentz, J.; Mounier, R.; Leclerc, J.; Treebak, J.T.; Pehmøller, C.; Sanz, N.; Sakakibara, I.; Saint-Amand, E.; Rimbaud, S. AMPK controls exercise endurance, mitochondrial oxidative capacity, and skeletal muscle integrity. *FASEB J.* **2014**, *28*, 3211–3224. [CrossRef]
60. Ju, J.-s.; Jeon, S.-i.; Park, J.-y.; Lee, J.-y.; Lee, S.-c.; Cho, K.-j.; Jeong, J.-m. Autophagy plays a role in skeletal muscle mitochondrial biogenesis in an endurance exercise-trained condition. *J. Physiol. Sci.* **2016**, *66*, 417–430. [CrossRef]
61. Lin, J.; Zhang, X.; Sun, Y.; Xu, H.; Li, N.; Wang, Y.; Tian, X.; Zhao, C.; Wang, B.; Zhu, B. Exercise ameliorates muscular excessive mitochondrial fission, insulin resistance and inflammation in diabetic rats via irisin/AMPK activation. *Sci. Rep.* **2024**, *14*, 10658. [CrossRef] [PubMed]
62. Jin, L.; Diaz-Canestro, C.; Wang, Y.; Tse, M.A.; Xu, A. Exerkines and cardiometabolic benefits of exercise: From bench to clinic. *EMBO Mol. Med.* **2024**, *16*, 432–444. [CrossRef] [PubMed]
63. Jia, D.; Hou, L.; Lv, Y.; Xi, L.; Tian, Z. Postinfarction exercise training alleviates cardiac dysfunction and adverse remodeling via mitochondrial biogenesis and SIRT1/PGC-1α/PI3K/Akt signaling. *J. Cell. Physiol.* **2019**, *234*, 23705–23718. [CrossRef] [PubMed]
64. Zhao, D.; Sun, Y.; Tan, Y.; Zhang, Z.; Hou, Z.; Gao, C.; Feng, P.; Zhang, X.; Yi, W.; Gao, F. Short-duration swimming exercise after myocardial infarction attenuates cardiac dysfunction and regulates mitochondrial quality control in aged mice. *Oxidative Med. Cell. Longev.* **2018**, *2018*, 4079041. [CrossRef]
65. Mendham, A.E.; Goedecke, J.H.; Zeng, Y.; Larsen, S.; George, C.; Hauksson, J.; Fortuin-de Smidt, M.C.; Chibalin, A.V.; Olsson, T.; Chorell, E. Exercise training improves mitochondrial respiration and is associated with an altered intramuscular phospholipid signature in women with obesity. *Diabetologia* **2021**, *64*, 1642–1659. [CrossRef]
66. Burtscher, J.; Soltany, A.; Visavadiya, N.P.; Burtscher, M.; Millet, G.P.; Khoramipour, K.; Khamoui, A.V. Mitochondrial stress and mitokines in aging. *Aging Cell* **2023**, *22*, e13770. [CrossRef]
67. Li, H.; Liu, G.; Wang, B.; Momeni, M.R. Exosomes and microRNAs as mediators of the exercise. *Eur. J. Med. Res.* **2025**, *30*, 38. [CrossRef]
68. Gaál, Z.; Fodor, J.; Oláh, T.; Szabó, I.G.; Balatoni, I.; Csernoch, L. Implication of microRNAs as messengers of exercise adaptation in junior female triathlonists. *Sci. Rep.* **2024**, *14*, 22858. [CrossRef]
69. Song, R.; Hu, X.-Q.; Zhang, L. Mitochondrial MiRNA in cardiovascular function and disease. *Cells* **2019**, *8*, 1475. [CrossRef]
70. Carrer, M.; Liu, N.; Grueter, C.E.; Williams, A.H.; Frisard, M.I.; Hulver, M.W.; Bassel-Duby, R.; Olson, E.N. Control of mitochondrial metabolism and systemic energy homeostasis by microRNAs 378 and 378. *Proc. Natl. Acad. Sci. USA* **2012**, *109*, 15330–15335. [CrossRef]
71. Yamamoto, H.; Morino, K.; Nishio, Y.; Ugi, S.; Yoshizaki, T.; Kashiwagi, A.; Maegawa, H. MicroRNA-494 regulates mitochondrial biogenesis in skeletal muscle through mitochondrial transcription factor A and Forkhead box j3. *Am. J. Physiol. Endocrinol. Metab.* **2012**, *303*, E1419–E1427. [CrossRef] [PubMed]
72. Nahálková, J. Focus on molecular functions of anti-aging deacetylase SIRT3. *Biochemistry* **2022**, *87*, 21–34. [CrossRef] [PubMed]
73. Geng, L.; Zhang, T.; Liu, W.; Chen, Y. miR-494-3p modulates the progression of in vitro and in vivo Parkinson's disease models by targeting SIRT3. *Neurosci. Lett.* **2018**, *675*, 23–30. [PubMed]
74. He, T.; Sha, J.; Hu, Y.; Shao, C.; Zhou, Y.; Chen, L.; Yao, J.; Gao, J. Single-Cell Sequencing Identifies the Crucial Role of Mitochondrial Fission-Fusion Balance in Cardiac Hypertrophy Progression. *bioRxiv* **2025**. [CrossRef]
75. Pribil Pardun, S.; Bhat, A.; Anderson, C.P.; Allen, M.F.; Bruening, W.; Jacob, J.; Pendyala, V.V.; Yu, L.; Bruett, T.; Zimmerman, M.C. Electrical Pulse Stimulation Protects C2C12 Myotubes against Hydrogen Peroxide-Induced Cytotoxicity via Nrf2/Antioxidant Pathway. *Antioxidants* **2024**, *13*, 716.
76. Hernandez, G.; Thornton, C.; Stotland, A.; Lui, D.; Sin, J.; Ramil, J.; Magee, N.; Andres, A.; Quarato, G.; Carreira, R.S. MitoTimer: A novel tool for monitoring mitochondrial turnover. *Autophagy* **2013**, *9*, 1852–1861.
77. Laker, R.C.; Xu, P.; Ryall, K.A.; Sujkowski, A.; Kenwood, B.M.; Chain, K.H.; Zhang, M.; Royal, M.A.; Hoehn, K.L.; Driscoll, M. A novel MitoTimer reporter gene for mitochondrial content, structure, stress, and damage in vivo. *J. Biol. Chem.* **2014**, *289*, 12005–12015.
78. Supervia, M.; Turk-Adawi, K.; Lopez-Jimenez, F.; Pesah, E.; Ding, R.; Britto, R.R.; Bjarnason-Wehrens, B.; Derman, W.; Abreu, A.; Babu, A.S. Nature of cardiac rehabilitation around the globe. *eClinicalMedicine* **2019**, *13*, 46–56. [CrossRef]

79. Maruf, F.A.; Mohammed, J. Unmet Needs for Cardiac Rehabilitation in Africa: A Perennial Gap in the Management of Individuals with Cardiac Diseases. *High Blood Press. Cardiovasc. Prev.* **2023**, *30*, 199–206. [CrossRef]
80. Dalal, J.J.; Almahmeed, W.; Krittayaphong, R.; Nicholls, S.J.; Soomro, K.; Yeo, K. Consensus recommendations of the Asia Pacific Cardiometabolic Consortium on Secondary Prevention Strategies in Myocardial Infarction: Recommendations on pharmacotherapy, lifestyle modification and cardiac rehabilitation. *J. Asian Pac. Soc. Cardiol.* **2023**, *2*, e01. [CrossRef]

MDPI AG
Grosspeteranlage 5
4052 Basel
Switzerland
Tel.: +41 61 683 77 34

Journal of Clinical Medicine Editorial Office
E-mail: jcm@mdpi.com
www.mdpi.com/journal/jcm

www.ingramcontent.com/pod-product-compliance
Lightning Source LLC
LaVergne TN
LVHW070446061126
851858LV00011B/171